Surgical Management of the Transgender Patient

Surgical Management of the Transgender Patient

LOREN S. SCHECHTER, MD, FACS
Plastic Surgeon
Morton Grove, Illinois, USA

ELSEVIER

ELSEVIER

1600 John F. Kennedy Blvd.
Ste 1800
Philadelphia, PA 19103-2899

Surgical Management of the Transgender Patient

ISBN: 978-0-323-48089-5

Notices

Knowledge and best practice in this field are constantly changing. As new research and experience broaden our understanding, changes in research methods, professional practices, or medical treatment may become necessary.

Practitioners and researchers must always rely on their own experience and knowledge in evaluating and using any information, methods, compounds, or experiments described herein. In using such information or methods they should be mindful of their own safety and the safety of others, including parties for whom they have a professional responsibility.

With respect to any drug or pharmaceutical products identified, readers are advised to check the most current information provided (i) on procedures featured or (ii) by the manufacturer of each product to be administered, to verify the recommended dose or formula, the method and duration of administration, and contraindications. It is the responsibility of practitioners, relying on their own experience and knowledge of their patients, to make diagnoses, to determine dosages and the best treatment for each individual patient, and to take all appropriate safety precautions.

To the fullest extent of the law, neither the Publisher nor the authors, contributors, or editors, assume any liability for any injury and/or damage to persons or property as a matter of products liability, negligence or otherwise, or from any use or operation of any methods, products, instructions, or ideas contained in the material herein.

Library of Congress Cataloging-in-Publication Data

A catalog record for this book is available from the Library of Congress

Content Strategist: Belinda Kuhn
Content Development Specialist: Devika Ponnambalam/Donald Mumford
Design Direction: Renee Duenow

Endsheet Illustration by Brittney Leeane Williams. Commissioned by Fred and Susan Novy. © Loren S. Schechter.
We thank Alexander L.S. Bernat for assistance with computer editing.

Working together
to grow libraries in
developing countries

www.elsevier.com • www.bookaid.org

To the individuals who have struggled to be themselves
and those who have helped them.

Contributors

The editor would like to acknowledge and offer grateful thanks for the input of all contributors, without whom this first edition would not have been possible.

NIKITA ABHYANKAR, MD
Urology Resident
University of Illinois at Chicago
Chicago, IL, USA

FREDERIC ETTNER, MD
Private Practice – Family Medicine
Lincolnwood, IL, USA

RANDI ETTNER, PhD
New Health Foundation Worldwide
Evanston, IL, USA

JAMISON GREEN, PhD, MFA
Adjunct Professor
California Institute of Integral Studies
President
World Professional Association for Transgender
Health (WPATH)
San Francisco, CA, USA

ERVIN KOCJANCIC, MD
Lawrence S. Ross Professor of Urology
Department of Urology
University of Illinois Hospital and Health Science
System
Chicago, IL, USA

SLAWOMIR MARECIK, MD
Associate Professor of Clinical Surgery
University of Illinois at Chicago College
of Medicine
Colorectal Surgeon
Advocate Lutheran General Hospital
Park Ridge, IL, USA

MICHAEL NOONE, MD
Assistant Clinical Professor of Obstetrics and
Gynecology
University of Illinois at College of Medicine
Chicago, IL, USA

REBECCA B. SCHECHTER, MD
Endocrinologist
Highland Park, IL, USA

LISA SIMONS, MD
Division of Adolescent Medicine
Ann & Robert H. Lurie Children's Hospital
of Chicago
Instructor of Pediatrics
Northwestern University Feinberg School
of Medicine
Chicago, IL, USA

VIN TANGPRICHA, MD, PhD
Associate Professor of Medicine
Division of Endocrinology, Metabolism and Lipids
Department of Medicine, Emory University and the
Atlanta VA Medical Center
Atlanta, GA, USA

Foreword

I am honored to write this foreword to this amazing book—a first of its kind. For many decades, I have been deeply concerned about the lack of well-qualified surgeons willing and able to perform gender-confirmation surgeries. The lack of systemized training has been very disconcerting. I have watched surgeons get into the field and struggle to learn their skill. They have certainly benefited from experienced surgeons sharing their knowledge, but mostly, people have had to learn these specialized surgical techniques on their own and without any textbook to guide them.

This textbook fills that void. It is also very timely, as World Professional Association for Transgender Health has initiated their Global Education Initiative with specific training for surgeons and their efforts to establish clinical competency standards. This book will be an essential tool in training the next generation of surgeons to learn the skills and techniques of gender-confirmation surgery. It is also timely given the greater demand for surgeries around the world as health ministries and health insurance companies have acknowledged the medical necessity of these procedures and have been willing to make these accessible to those who need them. This has opened the door to many people who simply did not have the means or resources to these life-saving and enhancing procedures. But, this has also created a demand that has outstripped the supply of well-trained surgeons. Training is urgently needed, and this book will be an essential guide to any surgeon wanting to develop these skills.

While there are many facets and approaches of treating individuals with gender dysphoria, surgical procedures have been proven to be one of the most effective and medically necessary treatments. A positive result for these individuals is dependent upon the quality of the surgical outcome. Thus, becoming a skilled surgeon is essential to patients' ability to achieve a lasting personal comfort with their gendered selves—allowing them to maximize their overall health, psychological well-being, and self-fulfillment.

Not only does this significantly impact the lives of many individuals but also is very gratifying work for the skilled surgeon.

Loren Schechter is one of world's leading experts in gender-confirmation surgery. He has benefited from his mentors, and now has assembled an outstanding group of contributing authors to share their knowledge, skills, and wisdom with others. Not only does this book clearly describe the surgical procedures but also is very clearly and vividly illustrated. The procedures are the best available in this emerging field, and this book will also allow for further development as individuals study these procedures and techniques.

The impact and importance of this book cannot be overestimated. This will be an essential resource not only for any clinician conducting this work but also for the interdisciplinary teams that are involved in the overall management of these patients. By raising the standard of training and education of these procedures, this is a true gift to the transgender community around the world who will benefit from them.

And, for many transgender individuals who are seeking surgical treatments, this is a very useful way for them to make informed decisions about the procedures they will want and to better understand realistic outcomes.

Loren Schechter has created this masterpiece, which is also a gift of love and generosity, to pass on what he and others have learned and make it much easier for those entering the field to become the very best at what they do.

Eli Coleman, PhD
Past President and Chair of the Standards of Care Revision Committee
The World Professional Association for Transgender Health Academic Chair in Sexual Health
Professor and Director
Program in Human Sexuality
University of Minnesota Medical School
Minneapolis, MN, USA

Preface

My interest in plastic surgery arose from the unique opportunity to apply my knowledge of anatomy, physiology, and wound healing in a creative manner so as to address a wide variety of conditions. The fields of reconstructive surgery and microsurgery appealed to me because they address anatomic functionality and aesthetic appearance, both of which greatly impact patients' quality of life. I have been lucky to work with a number of people who helped me spark my passion for furthering this field. I am particularly appreciative for my colleagues and friends, Drs. Randi and Fred Ettner, Dr. Stan Monstrey, Dr. Lawrence Gottlieb, and Dr. Rados Djinovic, whose support has helped to shape my career path.

As my surgical career evolved, so did society's understanding and perceptions of issues related to gender dysphoria. With that, an increasing number of individuals suffering from gender dysphoria began seeking gender confirming surgical therapies, and I became keenly aware of the surgical needs of this underserved community. These developments drove me to advance my understanding of the surgical management of transgender individuals.

While there is still work to be done, I am proud of the strides we have made in providing quality care to transgender individuals. The World Professional Association for Transgender Heath has been a leader in raising awareness and providing guidelines for transgender care. Brave individuals have stepped forward to fight for insurance coverage for gender confirming surgeries, leading to improved benefits from Medicare and other third party payers. Hospitals throughout the country are working to set up programs for transgender individuals. I feel privileged to be part of this progress.

While gender confirming surgery represents one of many therapies for transgender individuals with gender dysphoria, it can be pivotal in allowing individuals to become their true selves. This text represents an evolution of surgical techniques, as well as a framework around which surgical therapies are based to allow for these transformations. While techniques will continue to advance, an understanding of the surgical principles is fundamental to this process. I hope readers will learn about the challenges and complexities in the surgical care of transgender individuals, and, in doing so, will be inspired to work to further advance the quality of transgender care.

Loren S. Schechter, MD, FACS
Plastic Surgeon
Morton Grove, IL, USA

Contents

Surgical Management of the Transgender Patient

CHAPTER 1

Introduction

The surgical care of individuals suffering from gender dysphoria or gender incongruence has undergone rapid transformation over the last several years. Although not all individuals with gender dysphoria need or desire surgery, many do. With an increased recognition as to the importance of surgical therapy, coupled with improved access to care resulting from expanded insurance coverage, more individuals are seeking surgery.

My first experiences caring for transgender individuals occurred during my early years as a plastic surgery resident, under the mentorship of Dr Lawrence Gottlieb. Subsequently, when I entered practice, Drs Fred and Randi Ettner, experts in the medical and psychological care of transgender persons, approached me with the goal of offering surgical treatment options for their patients. As I became more involved with the surgical care and the advocacy efforts for transgender persons, I learned about the limited resources available to this population.

During my career, I have been fortunate to work with leaders around the world, including Professor Stan Monstrey and Rados Djinovic. In addition, I was able to draw on my experience from congenital, traumatic, and oncologic cases and develop and advance techniques for gender-confirming surgeries. As of the writing of this book, no formal surgical training programs exist. This surgical text is a first step in filling the educational gap. It is my hope that surgeons will gain experience in the field of gender surgery, thereby continuing to advance operative techniques.

This text outlines many surgical therapies (Box 1.1), but it must be taken in context. The care of individuals with gender dysphoria requires a multidisciplinary approach. Although surgery often represents the culmination of an individual's life journey, it is not undertaken in a vacuum. The surgeon must work collaboratively with mental health professionals, primary care physicians, endocrinologists, and other specialists.

BOX 1.1
Surgical treatment options

Surgical procedures for transwomen
- Vaginoplasty
  - Penile disassembly and inversion vaginoplasty
  - Intestinal vaginoplasty
- FFS (facial feminization surgery)
  - Brow lift (hair advancement)
  - Frontal bone reduction (burring vs osteoplastic ± onlay graft)
  - Mandible reduction (angle and/or chin)
  - Rhinoplasty
  - Malar implant
  - Lip shortening and/or augmentation
  - Hair transplantation
- Thyroid chondroplasty ("tracheal shave")
- Breast augmentation
- Body contouring

Surgical procedures for transmen
- Chest surgery
  - Limited incision
  - Circumareolar/vertical
  - Double incision
- Metoidioplasty
- Phalloplasty
  - Radial forearm flap
  - Anterolateral thigh flap
  - Musculocutaneous latissimus dorsi flap

CHAPTER 2

Background

DEFINITIONS

Gender Dysphoria

The term gender dysphoria describes a heterogeneous group of individuals who express varying degrees of discomfort with or disassociation from their anatomic gender. Some people with this condition, in order to manage the discrepancy or imbalance they experience, desire to possess the secondary sexual characteristics of the opposite sex.[1] Not all transgender persons have gender dysphoria. For those who do, medical and surgical therapy can play a pivotal role in relieving their psychological discomfort.[2–9]

Over the past several decades, there has been significant progress in the understanding and treatment of individuals suffering from gender dysphoria. In 1984, Dr Milton Edgerton noted that, "transsexualism is a severe, and pathologic condition that is undesirable for both the patient and society...and non-surgical treatment continues to be expensive, time-consuming, and enormously disappointing."[10] Much has changed since Edgerton's statement. Advances in the psychological, medical, and surgical care of individuals with gender dysphoria have resulted in a multidisciplinary approach, aimed at improved quality of life and destigmatization for this underserved and diverse population. In addition, social and political changes have raised awareness as to the importance of providing safe and affirming environments, free from discrimination. In 2010, The World Professional Association for Transgender Health (WPATH) released a statement calling for the de-psycho-pathologization of gender nonconformity, stating that, "the expression of gender characteristics, including identities, that are not stereotypically associated with one's assigned sex at birth is a common and culturally diverse human phenomenon [that] should not be judged as inherently pathologic or negative."[11]

WPATH developed the Standards of Care (SOC) to help provide "the highest standards" of care for transgender individuals. The SOC state that the overarching treatment goal is "...lasting personal comfort with the gendered self, in order to maximize overall health, psychological well-being and self-fulfillment."[12] Since WPATH published the first version of the SOC in 1979, the guidelines have been updated 6 times, reflecting increasing understanding of the transgender population and the delivery of optimal care.

Descriptions

Pyschosexual development and differentiation entails 3 major components:

- Gender identity, referring to one's sense of belonging to the male or female sex category, a combination of both, or neither, regardless of the sex assigned at birth;
- Gender role, sexually dimorphic behaviors and psychological characteristics within the population, such as toy preferences, clothing, and mannerisms; and
- Sexual orientation, one's pattern of erotic responsiveness as reflected in the sex of one's partner(s).

As noted by the Institute of Medicine's 2011 report on the health of lesbian, gay, bisexual, and transgender people, transgender individuals represent a diverse group of people who are defined according to their gender identity and presentation. This group includes persons whose gender identity differs from the sex originally assigned to them at birth or whose gender expression varies significantly from what is traditionally associated for that sex (ie, people identified as male at birth who are perceived as feminine and subsequently identify as female, and people identified as female at birth who appear more masculine and later identify as male). In addition, transgender persons may vary from or reject traditional cultural conceptualizations of gender in terms of the male-female dichotomy, or "binary." The Institute of Medicine's study also reported that the transgender population is varied in sexual expression and sexual orientation. Transgender people can be heterosexual, homosexual, or bisexual in their sexual orientation. Some lesbians, gay men, and bisexuals are transgender; most are not.[13]

Some transgender individuals have undergone medical interventions to alter their sexual anatomy and physiology; others wish to have such procedures in the future, and still others do not request medical or surgical intervention. In recent years, recognition that some individuals do not see themselves in the traditional male or female gender role has gained acceptance. Gender non-conforming or gender expansive describes a difference between an individual's gender identity, role, or expression and that of cultural norms. Some, but not all, gender-nonconforming individuals experience gender dysphoria.

EPIDEMIOLOGY

Although early estimates on the prevalence of gender dysphoria were focused on identification of individuals for gender confirmation surgery, it was later realized that some individuals neither desired, nor were candidates for, such surgery.[7,12] Early estimates of the prevalence of transsexualism were 1 in 37,000 biological males and 1 in 107,000 biological females.[14] Interestingly, approximately 3 times as many biological males as compared with biological females sought genital surgery. This historical discrepancy may exist for multiple reasons, including less accessibility, and more complicated—and expensive—surgical options available for biological females. However, with increased third-party coverage for gender confirmation surgery, there has been a corresponding increase in the number of biological females seeking genital surgery. More recent data estimate that 1 in 11,900 adult biological males and 1 in 30,400 adult biological females undergo genital procedures.[15]

The true prevalence of gender dysphoria is likely much greater than these early estimates. With increased advocacy, acceptance, and access to care, individuals are now able to seek medical attention in an atmosphere free from harassment or shame.

HISTORY

Transsexualism, gender dysphoria, and gender variance have been recorded throughout history and across cultures. These feelings have manifested as a spectrum of findings ranging from a conflict or feelings of inappropriateness of the assigned sex to a desire to surgically change one's external appearance. References to these conditions are included in, for example, the ancient Greek literature of Herodotus, the lives of the Roman emperors Caligula and Elagabalus, the literature of Shakespeare, and accounts of the French diplomat Chevalier d'Eon.[16]

In addition, the surgical alteration of one's genitalia has occurred for millennia. Eunuchs, or castrated men, have existed since Biblical times, and self-inflicted operations were described in

seventeenth century diaries as providing, "great and lasting subjective relief of gender dysphoria."[17] Moreover, in South Asia, the Hijra, or "third sex," are boys who undergo voluntary demasculinization surgery, often consisting of removal of the penis, testes, and scrotum. This surgery prevents the development of secondary sexual characteristics and maintains a childlike appearance.[18] Likewise, in Thailand, the Kathoey, sometimes referred to as ladyboys, may range from men who dress as women to what may more commonly be referred to as transgender.

In the modern medical sense, accounts of transsexualism were first mentioned in the German medical literature by Friedrich in 1830, followed by a description of a case of "transvestism" by Westphal in 1870.[19] However, it is Magnus Hirschfeld, a German physician and pioneer in the field of sexology, who is credited with the term "transsexualism," when he used the term seelischer transsexualismus or "psychic transsexualism" in 1923.[20] Hirschfeld founded the Institut fuer Sexualwissenschaft (Institute for Sexual Science) in Berlin in 1919 and was credited for referring the first male-to-female patient for surgery. In addition, Hirschfeld oversaw the initial surgical management of the Danish transgender woman, Lili Elbe, who traveled to Berlin for removal of her testicles in 1931. Elbe eventually succumbed following 5 surgical procedures, including failed ovarian and uterus transplants by the surgeon Kurt Warnekros at the Dresden Municipal Women's Clinic. It is Dr Felix Abraham, a German surgeon, who was the first to report and publish his experience with staged vaginoplasty on 2 patients, in 1931.[19] Abraham described the surgery as "...a kind of emergency surgery necessary to save patients from worse self-inflicted procedures."[21] The first documented female-to-male phalloplasty procedure was performed by renowned British surgeon Sir Harold Gillies in 1945.[22]

In 1949, David O. Cauldwell, an American physician, used the term "psychopathia transexualis" in describing an individual who desired to be a member of the opposite sex.[18] This was significant in delineating the difference between "transsexualism" and "transvestism." In this sense, transvestism was used to describe dressing or acting in a style typically associated with the "opposite sex." The contemporary study of transsexualism is credited to a public lecture and paper by Dr Harry Benjamin in 1953.[21,23] Benjamin (1885–1986), a German-born physician, who had met Magnus Hirschfeld while in Berlin, received his doctorate for a dissertation regarding tuberculosis. Dr Benjamin also had an interest in hormonal research and sexual medicine. Following a professional visit to the United States in 1913, Dr Benjamin's return to Germany was disrupted when the ship on which he was traveling was caught mid-Atlantic by the Royal Navy during the outbreak of World War I. Preferring to return to the United States rather than be treated as an enemy alien in a British internment camp, Dr Benjamin began practicing general medicine in New York in 1915. With his interest in sexual medicine, Dr Benjamin began treating transgender individuals. He believed in a physiologic basis of transsexualism, drawing the distinction between transsexualism and transvestism. The medical, legal, political, and social climate at this time was generally unaccepting of persons of nontraditional gender identity and sexual orientation. For example, wearing clothing of the opposite sex in public, male castration, and homosexuality were illegal. Medical treatments for such "disorders" often consisted of electroconvulsive therapy, lobotomy, and forced drugging. In 1966, Benjamin's book, The Transsexual Phenomenon, raised awareness of the potential benefits of sex reassignment surgery,[23] and, in 1979, The Harry Benjamin International Gender Dysphoria Association (now known as WPATH) was formed to further research in the subject and knowledge exchange among physicians and other physical and mental health care providers.

The case of Christine Jorgensen, an American who underwent surgery in Denmark in the 1950s, drew international attention to the field of transsexualism. The case was published in the Journal of the American Medical Association in 1953,[24] and the Danish physician Dr Christian Hamburger detailed the hormonal and surgical therapy provided to Ms Jorgensen. Following permission by the Danish Ministry of Justice, Ms Jorgensen underwent surgical castration and penile amputation. The following year, Ms Jorgensen requested removal of the "last visible remains of the detested masculinity" and underwent additional surgery to feminize her genitalia.[24] However, per the requests of the patient, no vaginoplasty was performed. Dr Hamburger concluded by stating that, "the goal was attained; by hormonal feminization and operative demasculinization the patient's soma harmonized with the pronounced feminine psyche."[24]

Other notable individuals include Dr Renée Richards, an American ophthalmologist and professional tennis player who underwent sex reassignment surgery in 1975. Following denial of entry into the 1976 US Open by the United States Tennis Association, she disputed the ban. In 1977, the New York Supreme Court ruled in her favor.

In the 1950s, Dr Georges Burou, a French gynecologist practicing in Casablanca at the Clinique du Parc, described the anteriorly pedicled penile skin flap inversion technique. Dr Borou is reported to have performed more than 3000 male-to-female sex reassignment procedures, some on famous female impersonators.[25]

In America, Dr Milton Edgerton is credited with establishing the first multidisciplinary center for care of the transgender patient. The Johns Hopkins University Gender Identity Clinic was formed in 1965 and was composed of representatives from psychiatry, psychology, plastic surgery, gynecology, urology, and endocrinology. This multidisciplinary clinic was important in establishing a method of preoperative evaluation and postoperative care.[26] This clinic allowed the health care team to evaluate lessons learned from the operative experience. In 1979, Dr Jon Meyer, a psychiatrist at Johns Hopkins University, and his colleagues published a follow-up study of 100 patients treated at the Hopkins Gender Identity Clinic. Of these patients, 34 underwent surgery and 66 did not. In this study, the investigators described 2 groups of patients: those individuals who will self-select for or against surgery. Interestingly, Meyer noted that in both groups, improvement was demonstrated over time. Furthermore, the study found that although sex reassignment surgery "confers no objective advantage in terms of social rehabilitation...it remains subjectively satisfying to those who have...undergone it."[27] This finding is consistent with the idea that not all individuals with gender dysphoria request surgery.

In 1969, additional centers were formed in the United States. These centers included the Stanford Medical Center under the guidance of Drs Norman Fisk and Donald Laub; Trinidad, Colorado under the leadership of Dr Stanley Biber; and Neenah, Wisconsin under the direction of Dr Eugene Schrang. In Europe, centers opened at the University Hospital of the Free University of Amsterdam under the leadership of Drs Louis Gooren, F.G. Bouman, Peggy Cohen-Kettenis, and J. Joris Hage; at the University Hospital of Ghont in Belgium under the direction of Drs Stan Monstrey and Griet DeCuypere; and in Belgrade, Serbia under the leadership of Dr Sava Perovic and his protégés, Drs Miro Djordjevic and Rados Djinovic. These esteemed and dedicated physicians have continued to advance the field of transgender medicine and surgery.

As a result of long-ongoing advocacy efforts, in May 2014, The US Department of Health and Human Services (HHS) repealed a 1989 decision declaring genital reconstruction surgeries for transsexualism "experimental." The previous exclusion of gender-confirming surgeries was based on a 1981 report stating that "the safety and effectiveness of trans-sexual surgery had not been proven."[28] In the May 2014 ruling, HHS ruled that "...new evidence indicates that the...rationale for considering the surgery experimental is not valid... [and] new evidence indicates that transsexual surgery is a safe and effective treatment option for transsexualism in appropriate cases."[28] Following this, access to care was opened for Medicare beneficiaries.

However, it is Caitlyn Jenner, formerly Bruce, who recently has done more to advance the cause of individuals suffering from gender dysphoria than any other single person. Jenner won the gold medal in the men's decathlon in the 1974 Olympics, giving her the unofficial title of the "world's greatest athlete." Jenner then went on to a successful career in TV and media, including starring in the reality show, "Keeping up with the Kardashians." In 2015, Jenner announced publicly she is transgender. The generally positive media coverage has served to raise awareness as to the challenges facing this population.

CAUSE

The cause of gender dysphoria remains unknown.[29] Research has investigated genetics, hormonal influences, family dynamics, and psychoanalytical observations as possible contributing causes.[1] Early theories were based largely on psychoanalytic contexts, followed by attempts to define transgenderism in a biological context. There are essentially 3 theories relating to the cause of transgenderism: a psychological or sociologic cause, a biological cause, or some combination thereof.

Psychoanalytic explanations have ranged from an inability to separate on the part of the mother and child,[30] psychotic disorders,[31] and an unconscious motivation to discard bad and aggressive features.[29,32] As such, psychoanalysts viewed gender confirmation surgery as "psychosurgery" and argued that treatment of transgenderism could only be achieved through psychoanalysis.[29]

Proponents of a biological explanation have examined a variety of theories, including anatomic differences in the brains of transgender individuals as well as hormonal influences on brain development at critical gestational stages. Early biologic theories, referred to as gender transposition, examined hormone-induced cephalic differentiation using radiographic brain imaging.[29] This concept

relied on the "default theory," which suggested in the absence of androgens, an embryo will feminize, and in the presence of androgens, testes develop.[33] However, many of these theories rested on extrapolation from animal studies. Subsequent research demonstrated important differences between hormone secretions in humans and animals.

Some of the most recent theories have focused attention on identifying genetic links to explain transgenderism. However, at this time, no genetic markers have been detected. Instead, studies have used differences in physical characteristics between transgender persons and nontransgender persons as indirect evidence of a genetic cause. These studies include such factors as the observation of a high prevalence of left-handedness in transgender individuals,[34] height differences between transwomen and nontransgender males,[35] the presence of an anomalous inframammary ligament in transmen,[36] a higher rate of polycystic ovaries in transmen,[37] and differences in bone proportion and fat distribution.[29] Still other researchers have examined autopsied brains of transfemales and noted differences in the hypothalamus, an area of the brain involved in sexual behavior. Genetic females and transfemales were found to have similar and smaller volumes of the central sulci of the stria terminalis compared with both homosexual and heterosexual males.[38]

Despite continued research in this area, it is also recognized that a spectrum of gender variance exists. Furthermore, both cultural and social constructs play a significant factor in gender role. For example, although most of the studies compare transgender individuals to nontransgender individuals, these studies do not account for biological explanations as to cross-dressing heterosexual males or children with a history of gender identity disorder who become gender-typical adults. As Dr Randi Ettner concludes, "...the etiology of transgenderism remains unknown. The goal of treatment, however, is known and is indisputable: to assist gender-variant patients who request medical interventions by providing state-of-the-art treatment."[29]

REFERENCES

1. Brown GR. A review of clinical approaches to gender dysphoria. J Clin Psychiatry 1990;51(2):57–64.
2. Monstrey S, Hoebeke P, Dhont M, et al. Surgical therapy in transsexual patients: a multi-disciplinary approach. Acta Chir Belg 2001;101(5):200–9.
3. Mate-Kole C, Freschi M, Robin A. A controlled study of psychological and social change after

surgical gender reassignment in selected male transsexuals. Br J Psychiatry 1990;157:261–4.

4. Imbimbo C, Verze P, Palmieri A, et al. A report from a single institute's 14-year experience in treatment of male-to-female transsexuals. J Sex Med 2009; 6(10):2736–45.

5. Weyers S, Elaut E, De Sutter P, et al. Long-term assessment of the physical, mental, and sexual health among transsexual women. J Sex Med 2009;6(3):752–60.

6. Vujovic S, Popovic S, Sbutega-Milosevic G, et al. Transsexualism in Serbia: a twenty-year follow-up study. J Sex Med 2009;6(4):1018–23.

7. Kockott G, Fahrner EM. Transsexuals who have not undergone surgery: a follow-up study. Arch Sex Behav 1987;16(6):511–22.

8. Johansson A, Sundbom E, Hojerback T, et al. A five-year follow-up study of Swedish adults with gender identity disorder. Arch Sex Behav 2010;39(6):1429–37.

9. Cohen-Kettenis P, Pfafflin F. Transgenderism and intersexuality in children and adolescence: making choices. Thousand Oaks (CA): Sage; 2003.

10. Edgerton MT. The role of surgery in the treatment of transsexualism. Ann Plast Surg 1984;13(6):473–81.

11. World Professional Association for Transgender Health press release May 26, 2010. Available at: http://www.wpath.org/uploaded_files/140/files/de-psychopathologisation 5-26-10 on letterhead.pdf. Accessed December 1, 2015.

12. World Professional Association for Transgender Health Standards of Care. Available at: http://www.wpath.org/uploaded_files/140/files/Standards of Care, V7 Full Book.pdf. 2012. Accessed December 1, 2015.

13. Institute of Medicine. The health of lesbian, gay, bisexual, and transgender people: building a foundation for better understanding. Washington, DC: The National Academies Press; 2011.

14. Roberto LG. Issues in diagnosis and treatment of transsexualism. Arch Sex Behav 1983;12(5):445–73.

15. Van Kesteren PJ, Gooren LJ, Megens JA. An epidemiological and demographic study of transsexuals in the Netherlands. Arch Sex Behav 1996;25(6):589–600.

16. Edgerton M, Knorr N, Callison J. The surgical treatment of transsexual patients. Plast Reconstr Surg 1970;45(1):38–46.

17. Monstrey S, Selvaggi G, Ceulemans P, et al. Surgery: male-to-female patient. In: Ettner R, Monstrey S, Eyler E, editors. Principles of transgender medicine and surgery. New York: Haworth Press; 2007. p. 106.

18. Cauldwell D. Psychopathia transsexualis. Sexology 1949;16:274.

19. Abraham F. Genitalumwandlungen an zwei mannlichen transvestite. Zeitschrift für Sexualwissenschaft und Sexualpolitik 1931;18:223–6.

20. Hirshfeld M. Die intersexuelle constitution. Jahrbuch fuer Sexuelle Zwischenstufen 1923;23:3–27.

21. Benjamin H. Transvestism and transsexualism. Int J Sexology 1953;7:12–4.

22. Gillies H, Harrison R.I Congenital absence of the penis with embryological considerations. Br J Plast Surg 1948;1:8.

23. Benjamin H. The transsexual phenomenon. New York: The Julian Press; 1966.

24. Hamburger C, Sturup GK, Dahl-Iversen E. Transvestism; hormonal, psychiatric, and surgical treatment. J Am Med Assoc 1953;152(5):391–6.

25. Reed HM. Aesthetic and functional male to female genital and perineal surgery: feminizing vaginoplasty. Semin Plast Surg 2011;25(2):163–74.

26. Hembree WC, Cohen-Kettenis P, Delemarre-van de Waal HA, et al. Endocrine treatment of transsexual persons: an Endocrine Society clinical practice guideline. J Clin Endocrinol Metab 2009;94(9): 3132–54.

27. Meyer JK, Reter DJ. Sex reassignment. Follow-up. Arch Gen Psychiatry 1979;36(9):1010–5.

28. Department of Health and Human Services. Departmental Appeals Board. Appellate Division. NCD140.3, Transsexual Surgery. Docket No. A-13–87. Decision No. 2576. May 30, 2014. Available at: www.hhs.gov/dab/decisions/dabdecisions/dab2576.pdf. Accessed July 18, 2016.

29. Ettner R. The etiology of transsexualism. New York: The Haworth Press; 2007.

30. Macvicar K. The transsexual wish in a psychotic character. Int J Psychoanal Psychother 1978;7: 354–65.

31. Socarides CW. Transsexualism and psychosis. Int J Psychoanal Psychother 1978;7:373–84.

32. Lothstein LM. Psychological testing with transsexuals: a 30-year review. J Pers Assess Oct 1984; 48(5):500–7.

33. Crews D. Animal sexuality. Sci Am 1994;270:108–14.

34. Watson DB, Coren S. Left-handedness in male-to-female transsexuals. JAMA 1992;267(10):1342.

35. Ettner R, Schacht M, Brown J, et al. Transsexualism: the phenotypic variable. Poster presented at the 15th International Symposium on Gender Dysphoria, Harry Benjamin International Gender Dysphoria Association. Vancouver (Canada), September 1997.

36. van Straalen WR, Hage JJ, Bloemena E. The inframammary ligament: myth or reality? Ann Plast Surg 1995;35(3):237–41.

37. Bosinski HA, Schroder I, Peter M, et al. Anthropometrical measurements and androgen levels in males, females, and hormonally untreated female-to-male transsexuals. Arch Sex Behav 1997;26(2): 143–57.

38. Zhou JN, Hofman MA, Gooren LJ, et al. A sex difference in the human brain and its relation to transsexuality. Nature 1995;378(6552):68–70.

CHAPTER 3

Medical Therapy

DIAGNOSIS

Transgender is not a formal diagnosis.[1] Transgender individuals possess persistent concerns, uncertainties, and questions about gender identity. These issues often become the most important aspect of their life and prevent the establishment of an unconflicted gender identity. These individuals have passed a clinical threshold.

When such an individual meets the specified criteria in one of the 2 official nomenclatures, *The International Classification of Diseases-10 (ICD-10)* or the *Diagnostic Statistical Manual of Mental Disorders (5th Edition) (DSM-5)*, they are diagnosed as having a gender identity disorder (GID) or gender dysphoria.

In 1994, the *Diagnostic and Statistical Manual of Mental Disorders (Fourth Edition) (DSM-IV)* committee replaced the diagnosis of "transsexualism" with "gender identity disorder." According to *DSM-IV*, individuals must demonstrate a strong and persistent cross-gender identification and a persistent discomfort with their sex or a sense of inappropriateness in the gender role of that sex.[2] In *DSM-5*, published in 2013, the term "gender identity disorder" was replaced with the term "gender dysphoria." The diagnosis of gender dysphoria requires a marked difference between the individual's expressed/experienced gender, and the gender others would assign him or her. This difference must be present for 6 months and cause clinically significant distress or impairment in social, occupational, or other important areas of functioning.[3]

The *ICD-10* provides 5 diagnoses for GIDs.[4] These diagnoses include Transsexualism (F64.0), Dual-Role Transvestism (F64.1), Gender Identity Disorder of Childhood (64.2), Other Gender Identity Disorders (F64.8), and Gender Identity Disorder, Unspecified.

Transsexualism has 3 criteria, as follows.

1. The desire to live and be accepted as a member of the opposite sex, usually accompanied by the wish to make his or her body as congruent as possible with the preferred sex through surgery and hormone treatment.
2. The transsexual identity has been present persistently for at least 2 years.
3. The disorder is not a symptom of another mental disorder or a chromosomal abnormality.

It is important to realize that the *DSM-V* and *ICD-10* are designed to guide research and treatment. The designation of GID or gender dysphoria as mental disorders is not a license for stigmatization or for the deprivation of gender patients' civil rights.[1] In order to gain and maintain access to medical treatments, individuals often need a diagnosis. The change from "disorder" to "dysphoria" is designed to facilitate access to care without stigmatization.

HORMONAL THERAPY

Many persons with gender dysphoria desire hormone therapy in order to transition, and endocrinologists or primary care providers typically guide treatment (Table 3.1). Endocrine therapy can help relieve psychosocial discomfort by inhibiting the effects of endogenous hormones and inducing feminizing or masculinizing changes. As with surgery, hormone therapy requires a tailored approach. The administration of hormones is individualized based on the person's goals. Some people seek maximum feminization or masculinization, whereas others experience relief with an androgynous presentation resulting from hormonal minimization of existing secondary sex characteristics.[5]

Not all gender surgeries (ie, chest surgery) require preoperative hormone therapy. However, third-party payers often require documentation of duration of hormone therapy, or an explanation as to why a patient does not take hormones, before providing insurance approval for surgery.

Although specific hormonal regimens may vary between centers, the surgeon should be familiar with the possible side effects of hormonal therapy and how they relate to the surgical care of the transgender patient. These possible side effects include issues related to liver function, risk of venous thromboembolism, electrolyte imbalance, drug-drug interactions, and possible malignancy (ie, breast cancer).

The goal of endocrine therapy is to change secondary sex characteristics in order to reduce gender dysphoria and/or facilitate a physical presentation consistent with the individual's sense of self.[6] Hormonal therapy should be individualized to the needs and desires of patients, based on their goals and associated

TABLE 3.1 Hormonal therapies for transwomen and transmen		
Hormone therapies for transwomen		
Estrogens	Oral	
	17-β estradiol	2–6 mg daily
	Ethinyl estradiol	2–6 mg daily
	Conjugated estrogen	2.5–7.5 mg daily
	Transdermal	
	Estradiol patch	0.1–0.4 mg twice weekly
	Estradiol gel	0.1–0.4 mg daily
	Parenteral	
	Estradiol valerate or cypionate	5–20 mg IM every 2 wk or 2–10 mg IM weekly
Antiandrogens	Spironolactone	100–400 mg PO daily, divided doses
	Cyproterone acetate[a]	50–100 mg PO daily
	GnRH agonists	3.75 mg subcutaneous monthly
5-α reductase inhibitors	Finasteride	2.5 mg PO daily
	Dutasteride	0.5 mg PO every other day
Hormone therapies for transmen		
Testosterones	Oral	
	Testosterone undecanoate[a]	160–240 mg/d
	Transdermal	
	Testosterone patch	2.5–7.5 mg/d
	Testosterone 1% gel	2.5–10 mg/d
	Parenteral	
	Testosterone cypionate or enanthate	50–200 mg IM weekly or 100–200 mg every 2 wk
	Testosterone undecanoate	1000 mg IM every 10 wk

Abbreviations: IM, intramuscular; PO, by mouth.
[a] Not available in the United States.
Data from Hembree WC, Cohen-Kettenis P, Delemarre-van de Waal HA, et al. Endocrine treatment of transsexual persons: an Endocrine Society clinical practice guideline. J Clin Endocrinol Metab 2009;94(9):3132–54; Dr Fred Ettner, personal communication, April 2016; and Gardner IH, Safer JD. Progress on the road to better medical care for transgender patients. Curr Opin Endocrinol Diabetes Obes 2013;20(6):553–8.

medical conditions. Before initiating hormone therapy, a psychosocial assessment by a qualified mental health or medical practitioner should be performed. The Standards of Care (SOC) indicate the physician prescribing the hormones should[1]

1. Perform an initial evaluation that includes health history, physical examination, and relevant laboratory tests
2. Explain what feminizing/masculinizing medications do and the possible side effects/health risks (including the effects on fertility)
3. Confirm that the patient has the capacity to understand the risks and benefits of treatment and to make an informed decision about medical care
4. Inform the patient of the SOC and eligibility/readiness requirements
5. Provide ongoing medical monitoring, including regular physical and laboratory examination to monitor hormone effects and side effects.

Hormone Therapy for Transwomen

Feminization through hormonal therapy is achieved by 2 mechanisms: suppression of androgen effects and induction of female physical characteristics. Androgen suppression is achieved by using medications that either suppress gonadotropin-releasing hormone (GnRH) or are GnRH antagonists (progestational agents), suppress the production of luteinizing hormone (progestational agents, cyproterone acetate), interfere with testosterone production or metabolism of testosterone to dihydrotestosterone (spironolactone, finasteride, cyproterone acetate), or interfere with the binding of androgen to its receptors in target tissues (spironolactone, cyproterone acetate, flutamide). In addition, estrogen is used to induce female secondary sex characteristics, and its mechanism of action is through direct stimulation of receptors in target tissues.

Estrogens can be taken orally, intramuscularly, or cutaneously. Oral estrogens have the advantage of being inexpensive, widely available, and easy to administer. Oral estradiol is the preferred form of estrogen because it allows for straightforward measurement of serum estradiol concentration as a marker of efficacy. Other oral forms of estrogen include conjugated estrogens, such as Premarin, and synthetic estrogens, such as ethinyl estradiol. Importantly, use of oral estrogen, and specifically ethinyl estradiol, appears to increase the risk of venous thromboembolism. Intramuscular estrogens, such as estradiol valerate, can be taken every 1 to 2 weeks but can result in supraphysiologic levels of estradiol if serum levels are not properly monitored. Furthermore, many individuals find intramuscular injections inconvenient for long-term use. Cutaneous forms of estrogen, such as estradiol gel or estradiol patches, are also available and should be considered in patients with risk factors for venous thromboembolism. Cutaneous forms of estrogen have the disadvantage of more limited availability, increased cost, and potential adverse skin reactions.

Antiandrogens are often necessary as an adjunctive therapy to further reduce testosterone concentrations into the female range of less than 50 ng/mL. Spironolactone is the most commonly prescribed antiandrogen in the United States. Typical doses range from 100 to 400 mg daily in divided dosages. Cyproterone acetate, another commonly prescribed antiandrogen available in Europe and Canada, is not approved in the United States due to concerns with hepatotoxicity. This agent may have the additional advantage of having some progestin-like activity. Finally, 5-α reductase inhibitors (finasteride and dutasteride) block the conversion of testosterone to the more active agent, 5-α-dihydrotestosterone. These medications have beneficial effects on scalp hair loss, body hair growth, sebaceous glands, and skin consistency.

Progesterones can also be prescribed for transwomen. However, there is limited evidence that they offer any additional benefit in feminization of the body. In addition, because these agents may increase the risk of cerebrovascular disease, they are not routinely prescribed as part of the initial hormone regimen.

Within the first 6 months of therapy, there is typically a redistribution of body fat, decreased muscle mass, softening of skin, and decreased libido. Breast growth may be expected after 3 to 6 months of therapy and may continue for up to 2 years. Over a period of several years, body fat and facial hair become finer, although they are not completely eliminated by hormonal therapy alone. Progression of male pattern baldness may slow; however, hair does not typically regrow in bald areas. Many of the changes, perhaps with the exception of breast growth, are reversible with cessation of therapy.[6]

Although there are many beneficial effects of hormone therapy, there are also potential risks. These potential risks include an increased risk of venous thromboembolism, weight gain, hypertriglyceridemia, gallstones, and elevated liver enzymes. Other possible risks include cardiovascular disease, hypertension, hyperprolactinemia, and diabetes. The risk of breast cancer is, as of yet, indeterminate.

While on hormone therapy, transwomen should undergo routine laboratory assessment to confirm that their dosing provides therapeutic and not supraphysiologic concentrations of estradiol. The risk of adverse events increases with higher doses, particularly doses resulting in supraphysiologic levels of estradiol.[7] Optimal serum levels range from 100 to 300 pg/mL and should not exceed 400 pg/mL. In addition, electrolytes should be measured for those individuals on spironolactone, and testosterone should be measured to confirm that levels are in the female range.

Before gender confirmation surgery, patients should have their estradiol concentration measured in order to confirm that serum levels of estradiol are not supraphysiologic. Estrogen medication should be discontinued 2 weeks before surgery to reduce the risk of venous thromboembolism, and patients should be ambulatory before restarting estrogen therapy. Following orchiectomy, spironolactone can be discontinued, and estrogen doses may be lowered while still maintaining therapeutic concentrations of serum estradiol.

Hormone Therapy for Transmen

Masculinization through hormonal therapy for transmen follows general principles of hormone replacement for treatment of male hypogonadism. Both intramuscular and transdermal testosterone preparations are available and may be used to achieve testosterone values in the normal male range.[7] Testosterone therapy results in increased muscle mass and decreased fat mass, increased facial hair and acne, male pattern baldness, and increased libido. In addition, testosterone results in clitoromegaly, temporary or permanent decreased fertility, deepened voice, vaginal atrophy, and cessation of menses. If uterine bleeding does not cease, GnRH analogues or depot medroxyprogesterone may be added to stop menses and to reduce estrogen levels to those found in biological males.[7]

Transmen often prefer testosterone injections for their affordability, wide availability, and convenient schedule (every 1–2 weeks). However, some patients find the deep intramuscular injections painful. Testosterone undecanoate, a new intramuscular testosterone, can be taken less frequently (every 10 weeks) and was approved by the US Food and Drug Administration in 2014. However, warnings about pulmonary oil microembolism with this testosterone preparation have limited its use in the United States.

Testosterone patches or gels are good options for transmen but are also more expensive than intramuscular testosterone and require daily application. Skin irritation is often reported with patches, and gels carry the risk of transfer of testosterone to women or children in close contact. Subcutaneous testosterone pellets are another option for testosterone therapy, but they require a minor surgical procedure every 12 weeks.

Ideally, testosterone administered intramuscularly should be measured at the peak and trough to ensure that serum concentrations are in the therapeutic range (typically 400–1000 ng/mL). Timing for checking levels is less critical for patients on patches or gel, provided they are compliant with therapy. Complete blood count (CBC) and liver function level should be monitored because testosterone therapy can result in erythrocytosis and elevation in liver enzymes. Other risks of testosterone therapy include hypertension, excessive weight gain, salt retention, lipid changes, cystic acne, and adverse psychological changes.[7]

Preoperatively, transmen should discontinue their testosterone 2 weeks before gender confirmation surgery. The risk of postoperative venous thromboembolism is lower than in a transwoman. However, testosterone can be converted to estradiol in adipose tissue by the aromatase enzyme, especially when present in high concentrations. Patients should not restart their testosterone therapy until they are ambulatory after surgery.

PRIMARY AND PREVENTATIVE CARE

Preventative health care of the transgender individual includes clinical and laboratory monitoring and allows assessment of the beneficial effects associated with hormonal therapy as well as the possible adverse reactions. Monitoring of weight and blood pressure, directed physical examinations, CBCs, renal and liver function tests, and lipid and glucose measurements should be considered.

Additional tests for transwomen on estrogen therapy include measurement of prolactin levels, evaluation for cardiac risk factors, screening for prostate disease as recommended for biological men, and screening for breast cancer as recommended for biological women.[7]

For transmen, evaluation of bone mineral density should be performed if risk factors for osteoporosis are present. In addition, if mastectomy, hysterectomy, oophorectomy are not completed, mammograms and annual Papanicolaou smear, as recommended by the American Cancer Society and American College of Obstetricians and Gynecologists, respectively, should be considered.[7]

ADOLESCENT THERAPY

Over the past decade, an emerging area of clinical interest involves the treatment of transgender adolescents. Although gender identity in early childhood can be dynamic and changing, gender identity affirmed during adolescence may predict gender identity that persists into adulthood.[8] Adolescents with gender dysphoria may find the physical changes of puberty unbearable. These changes may result in depression, anxiety, social withdrawal, self-harming behavior, substance abuse, and in some cases, suicide.[9,10]

Increasing numbers of gender-nonconforming adolescents are presenting for care at earlier ages.[11–13] Early access to care for these adolescents may prevent or alleviate psychological suffering. Although management may vary among clinics, consensus supports a multidisciplinary approach to care ideally delivered by a combination of medical and mental health professionals with gender-related expertise and knowledge of child and adolescent development. A growing number of multidisciplinary centers in the United States embrace an affirming philosophy of care that views gender identity as a spectrum rather than binary and, as such, refrain from interpreting gender nonconformity as an abnormal human experience. Affirming approaches do not presume a specific gender identity but allow youth to safely explore and affirm their own sense of self, while supporting them living as they feel most comfortably in the world.

Both the Endocrine Society and the World Professional Association for Transgender Health have published guidelines for the treatment of transgender adolescents.[1,7] However, care should be designed to meet the unique needs of each adolescent and should be based on the presence or absence of gender dysphoria. The extent to which an individual requires either medical or mental health treatment can vary widely. Importantly, similar to transgender adults, not all gender-nonconforming or transgender adolescents desire to transition socially, medically, or surgically. Goals for treatment of adolescents include increasing self-esteem, improving social and academic functioning, and providing support for their families and community.

Pubertal suppression and cross-sex hormones are 2 forms of hormonal intervention that may be considered for gender dysphoric peripubertal and pubertal youth, respectively. Current guidelines recommend that all adolescents considering hormonal interventions first meet with a mental health professional. The mental health provider should explore gender dysphoria, identify and treat coexisting mental health concerns, and assess psychosocial support.[1,7] In addition, mental health providers should also educate and counsel families about the course of gender dysphoria in adolescents, treatment approaches, and confirm understanding of the expected physical effects, side effects, and risks of the desired medical intervention.[13]

The physical changes of puberty result from maturation of the hypothalamopituitarygonadal axis and development of secondary sex characteristics. In female adolescents, the first physical sign of puberty is breast budding, whereas in male adolescents, an increase in testicular volume heralds the onset of puberty (Fig. 3.1). The experience of puberty provokes intense distress for many gender-nonconforming adolescents. For some youth, gender dysphoria emerges at puberty. Pubertal suppression with GnRH agonists, a fully reversible medical intervention, may be beneficial for some youth. These agonists suppress the production of endogenous sex steroids by blocking GnRH stimulation of the pituitary gland, thereby suppressing production of gonadotropins. When administered early, GnRH agonists may prevent the development of secondary sex characteristics of an undesired puberty, some of which are irreversible (eg, voice deepening, laryngeal prominence development, breast development) and may improve physical outcome for those adolescents with persistent gender dysphoria who, ultimately, transition with cross-sex hormones. Treatment with GnRH agonists may alleviate psychological distress related to pubertal development, thereby allowing youth an opportunity to engage in gender exploration without the ongoing worry about their bodies changing. This opportunity is especially critical for adolescents who have just begun to question their gender. Finally, pubertal suppression affords adolescents and families more time for learning, counseling,

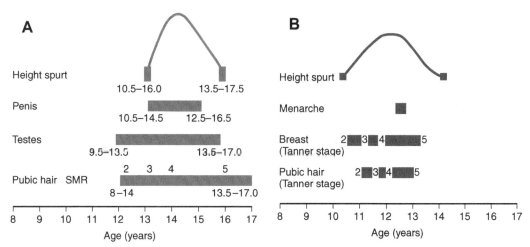

Fig. 3.1 (A) Age at time of physiologic changes during natal female and natal male puberty. (B) Sequence of pubertal events in the average American girl. SMR, sexual maturity rating. ([A] Adapted from Tanner JM. Growth at adolescence. Oxford: Blackwell Scientific Publications; 1962; and [B] From Tanner JM. Growth and endocrinology of the adolescent. In: Gardner LI, editor. Endocrine and genetic diseases of childhood and adolescents. 2nd edition. Philadelphia: WB Saunders; 1975.)

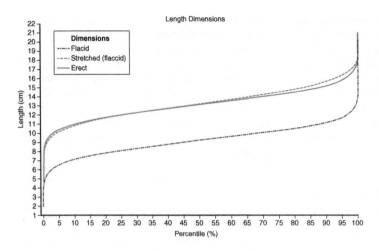

Fig. 3.2 Length of erect phallus. The dimensions of the natal, adult male phallus are helpful in guiding not only phalloplasty procedures but also constructing a functional vagina of adequate proportions in order to allow intercourse. If, as a result of pubertal suppression, full penile development is not realized, alternatives to penile inversion vaginoplasty (ie, intestinal vaginoplasty) will be necessary. (*From* Veale D, Miles S, Bramley S, et al. Am I normal? A systematic review and construction of nomograms for flaccid and erect penis length and circumference in up to 15,521 men. BJU Int 2015; 115(6):978–86; with permission.)

and decision-making. The Endocrine Society guidelines recommend that GnRH agonists may be started for gender-nonconforming youth no earlier than Tanner Stage 2.[7]

For adolescents with persistent gender dysphoria, treatments such as estrogen and testosterone therapy may be administered to facilitate an appearance that is more congruent with the adolescent's experienced gender. Estrogen and sometimes androgen-blocking medications such as spironolactone (for those not using GnRH agonists) may be used for feminization, and testosterone may be used for masculinization. These hormones are considered partially reversible treatments because they induce some changes that are reversible and others that are not. The Endocrine Society guidelines outline readiness and eligibility criteria for starting cross-sex hormones. Although the current version of the guidelines recommends that sex hormones may be started at age 16, some clinics in the United States start hormone therapy earlier with the goal of providing peer-concordant puberty.[7] As with pubertal suppression, adolescents seeking hormonal intervention must be capable of providing consent and have the support of legal guardians.

Hormone-treated adolescents may be referred for surgery when they are satisfied with the hormonal effects and social role change, and they desire definitive surgical changes.[7] Surgery is typically considered at 18 years of age, although individual exceptions, especially for chest surgery in transmales, may be appropriate.

From a surgical standpoint, one of the advantages of pubertal suppression may be less invasive surgical procedures (ie, limited-incision chest surgery as opposed to double-incision chest surgery

with free nipple grafts) or even the ability to forego certain procedures (ie, facial feminization). However, one potential drawback is the need to develop alternate surgical techniques for genital reconstruction, especially in transwomen. If, as a result of pubertal suppression, full penile length is not realized, alternate methodologies (ie, intestinal vaginoplasty) may be required in order to construct a functional vagina (Fig. 3.2).

The need for medical care for gender-nonconforming adolescents has only recently been recognized in the United States. A growing number of multidisciplinary gender clinics are beginning to expand the scope of services offered to adolescents to include options such as fertility-preservation counseling and services, gender-confirming surgery, voice training, and support groups for adolescents and parents. Long-term follow-up studies are needed to examine the impact of this care on the psychological well-being of gender-nonconforming adolescents with gender dysphoria.

REFERENCES

1. World Professional Association for Transgender Health Standards of Care. Available at: http://www.wpath.org/uploaded_files/140/files/Standards of Care, V7 Full Book.pdf. Accessed December 1, 2015.
2. American Psychiatric Association. Diagnostic and statistical manual of mental disorders: DSM-IV. 4th edition. Washington, DC: American Psychiatric Association; 1994.
3. American Psychiatric Association. Diagnostic and statistical manual of mental disorders. 5th edition. Washington, DC: American Psychiatric Association; 2013.

4. World Health Organization. The ICD-10 classification of mental and behavioural disorders: clinical descriptions and diagnostic guidelines. Geneva (Switzerland): World Health Organization; 1992.

5. Factor RJ, Rothblum ED. Exploring gender identity and community among three groups of transgender individuals in the United States: MTFs, FTMs, and genderqueers. Health Sociol Rev 2009; 17:241–59.

6. Dahl M, Feldman J, Goldberg J, et al. Physical aspects of transgender endocrine therapy. Int J Transgenderism 2006;9(3–4):111–34.

7. Hembree WC, Cohen-Kettenis P, Delemarre-van de Waal HA, et al. Endocrine treatment of transsexual persons: an Endocrine Society clinical practice guideline. J Clin Endocrinol Metab 2009;94(9): 3132–54.

8. Steensma TD, McGuire JK, Kreukels BP, et al. Factors associated with desistence and persistence of childhood gender dysphoria: a quantitative follow-up study. J Am Acad Child Adolesc Psychiatry 2013;52(6):582–90.

9. Bonifacio HJ, Rosenthal SM. Gender variance and dysphoria in children and adolescents. Pediatr Clin North Am 2015;62(4):1001–16.

10. Reisner SL, Vetters R, Leclerc M, et al. Mental health of transgender youth in care at an adolescent urban community health center: a matched retrospective cohort study. J Adolesc Health 2015;56(3):274–9.

11. de Vries AL, Steensma TD, Doreleijers TA, et al. Puberty suppression in adolescents with gender identity disorder: a prospective follow-up study. J Sex Med 2011;8(8):2276–83.

12. Wood H, Sasaki S, Bradley SJ, et al. Patterns of referral to a gender identity service for children and adolescents (1976–2011): age, sex ratio, and sexual orientation. J Sex Marital Ther 2013;39:1–6.

13. Spack NP, Edwards-Leeper L, Feldman HA, et al. Children and adolescents with gender identity disorder referred to a pediatric medical center. Pediatrics 2012;129(3):418–25.

CHAPTER 4

Surgical Therapy

EMBRYOLOGY

Genetic sex is determined at fertilization, either XX or XY. For the first 6 weeks of development, gender is not distinguishable, and this is known as the indifferent period. Characteristic external genitalia begin forming about the ninth week of gestation.

Sexual differentiation of the internal and external female genitalia requires no active intervention or ovarian activity; it is considered the default pathway. However, androgen production by the Leydig cells and Mullerian inhibiting hormone (MIH) production by the Sertoli cells are required for the development of the male external genitalia.

The internal genitalia can only develop into one gender and are termed "unipotent." In the male, the Wolffian ducts develop from the mesonephric ducts, and in the female, the Mullerian ducts develop from the paramesonephric ducts. In the male, MIH and androgens prevent development of female internal genitalia. In addition, androgens actively maintain the Wolffian ducts, whereas MIH induces the regression of the Mullerian ducts. In the female, Wolffian ducts regress in the absence of androgens (Fig. 4.1).

External genitalia have the potential to be either male or female and are termed "bipotential." In order to develop male external genitalia, androgens are required. In both sexes, in about the fourth week of development, the genital tubercle elongates to form the phallus. In a developing male, androgens induce the fusion of the urethral folds to form the urethra. In addition, the genital tubercle enlarges to form the glans penis, and midline fusion of the genital swellings results in formation of the scrotum. In the female, the urethral folds and genital swellings remain separate and form the labia minora and majora. The genital tubercle forms the clitoris.

From the author's perspective, in constructing the appropriate physical morphology, the relevant homologous structures are used to create "like-with-like." This philosophy forms the foundation on which he has developed his surgical techniques.

GOALS OF SURGICAL THERAPY

Congruent Genitalia

As described in the Standards of Care (SOC), the overarching treatment goal for transgender individuals is to maximize health, well-being, and fulfillment (Figs. 4.2 and 4.3).[1] Toward this end, gender confirmation surgery can provide the appropriate physical morphology and alleviate the extreme psychological discomfort that many patients experience.[2-6] Furthermore, as discussed by Meyer in 2001[7] and Cohen-Kettenis and Kuiper[8] in 1984, adjusting the mind to the body is not an effective treatment, while adjusting the body to the mind is the best way to assist severely gender dysphoric persons.

Congruent genitalia can allow an individual to experience harmony between one's body and self-identity, appear nude in social situations without violating taboos (ie, bathrooms, locker rooms, physician offices), and, in some states, have legal identification concordant with their physical appearance.[1]

Surgical goals for transwomen

Vaginoplasty. A successful surgical result involves the creation of a natural-appearing vagina and mons pubis[9] that are sensate and functional, including removal of the stigmatizing scrotum, creation of feminine-appearing labia majora and minora, construction of a sensate neoclitoris, and development of adequate vaginal depth and introital width for intercourse. Additional desirable qualities include a smooth, graded, and contiguous appearance to the labia majora, a moist appearance to the labia minora simulating the vestibular lining in natal females, clitoral hooding, and lubrication for intercourse (Box 4.1, Fig. 4.4).

Ancillary procedures. Aside from genital reconstruction, *breast augmentation*, *thyroid chondroplasty* ("tracheal shave"), *facial feminization*, and *body contouring* offer additional procedures designed to feminize one's appearance (Figs. 4.5 and 4.6).

Surgical goals for transmen

Chest surgery. This procedure, commonly performed before genital surgery, involves bilateral subcutaneous mastectomies, liposuction of the chest, and repositioning and resizing of the nipple-areola complex, when necessary. Several different techniques are used, and the choice of technique depends on the volume of breast parenchyma, degree of breast ptosis, position and

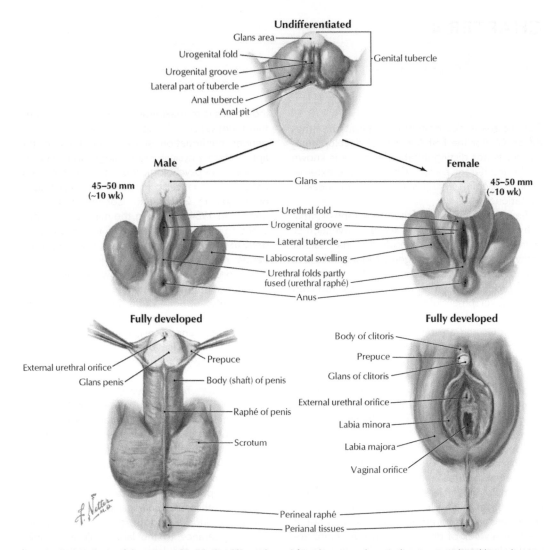

Fig. 4.1 Embryology of the external genitalia. The male and female external genitalia are considered homologous structures, that is, there is a corresponding anatomic part in each of the biological sexes. In transwomen, the component parts of the male anatomy are reassembled in order to construct the relevant female anatomy (mons pubis, vagina, clitoris, urethra, and labia minora). Conversely, in transmen, the female anatomy is removed and reassembled in order to construct portions of the male anatomy (scrotum and membranous urethra). For the patient undergoing metoidioplasty, the local anatomic structures will suffice in creating the phallus. However, in those individuals requesting phalloplasty, the use of remote tissue is required. (Copyright © 2016. Used with permission of Elsevier. All rights reserved. www.netterimages.com.)

size of the nipple-areola complex, and degree of skin elasticity (Box 4.2, Fig. 4.7).

Metoidioplasty. This procedure entails lengthening of the virilized clitoris. It can be performed with urethral lengthening, thereby allowing for urination while standing (Fig. 4.8).

Phalloplasty. As outlined by Professor Stan Monstrey and colleagues,[10] an ideal phallic reconstruction should result in an aesthetic phallus with both tactile and erogenous sensation, the ability to

void while standing, minimal morbidity of the surgical intervention and donor site, an aesthetic scrotum, and the ability to experience sexual satisfaction postoperatively (Box 4.3).

Although phalloplasty (Fig. 4.9) represents the most complete genitoperineal transformation, it requires complex, staged procedures, the use of tissue from remote sites, and the risk of complications associated with urethral reconstruction and implantable prostheses. For these reasons, some individuals forego phalloplasty and choose metoidioplasty instead.

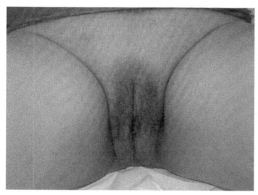

Fig. 4.2 Postoperative vaginoplasty, performed with penile disassembly and inversion technique, demonstrating the mons pubis (fatty tissue overlying pubic bone, including the vulva and labia majora). Note the smooth, graded, and contiguous appearance to the labia majora.

BOX 4.1
Criteria for an aesthetic and functional vaginoplasty

- Removal of the scrotum
- Feminine-appearing labia majora
  - Smooth, graded, and contiguous appearance
- Feminine-appearing labia minora
  - Moist appearance simulating the vestibular lining
- Sensate neoclitoris with clitoral hood
- Adequate vaginal depth and width for intercourse

Goals for nonconforming individuals

For individuals who do not belong to traditional male and female gender roles, varying degrees of hormone therapy and surgical intervention may be appropriate. Importantly, a treatment plan should be tailored to meet the goals of each individual.

MULTIDISCIPLINARY TREATMENT

Although the goals of surgery include a successful cosmetic and functional result with minimal complications, surgery is only one determinant in the overall therapeutic process.[11] The surgeon is part of a health care team that includes mental health professionals, primary care providers, endocrinologists, and midlevel practitioners. As such, the surgeon performing gender confirmation procedures must assume an active and integral role in the overall care of the patient. It is the responsibility of the operating surgeon to understand the diagnosis that has led to the recommendation for surgery, medical comorbidities that may impact the surgical outcome, the effects of hormonal therapy on the patient's health, and the patient's ultimate satisfaction with the surgical result.[12] Furthermore, the surgeon should assist with the coordination of

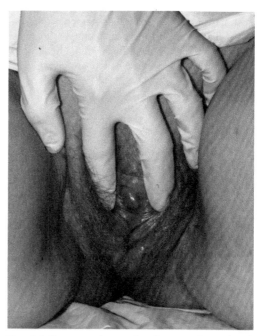

Fig. 4.4 Postoperative vaginoplasty performed with penile disassembly and inversion technique. The neoclitoris is formed from the dorsal glans penis; the vaginal lining is formed from penile and scrotal-perineal flaps, and the urethra is shortened, spatulated, and used for creation of the labia minora and vestibular lining.

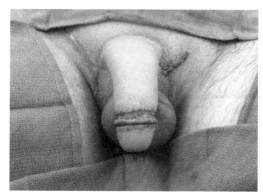

Fig. 4.3 Postoperative phalloplasty performed with radial forearm flap. The procedure includes glansplasty, scrotoplasty, and secondary placement of testicular implants.

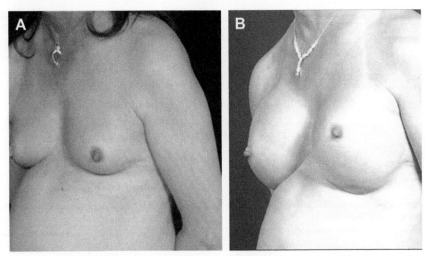

Fig. 4.5 (A) Preoperative photograph. Breast augmentation in a transwoman using silicone gel implants placed in a subpectoral pocket through an inframammary crease incision. (B) Postoperative photograph.

the patient's postoperative care in order to assure continuity.

Recognizing that, in appropriately selected individuals, gender confirmation surgery is the best way to normalize the lives of transgender persons,[13] the question of how best to integrate the surgeon in the multidisciplinary team continues to evolve. Although typically introduced to the patient only after diagnosis and hormonal therapy, the surgeon must actively participate in understanding the patient's diagnosis and medical therapies. In order to do so, a collaborative effort with the health care

team is recommended. Understanding the limitations in access to formal multidisciplinary gender teams, the World Professional Association for Transgender Health SOC provides recommendations designed to standardize the process of surgical evaluation, treatment, and postoperative care of transgender individuals.[1] The goal of this standardized approach to surgical management is to lead to uniform and consistent surgical results worldwide.

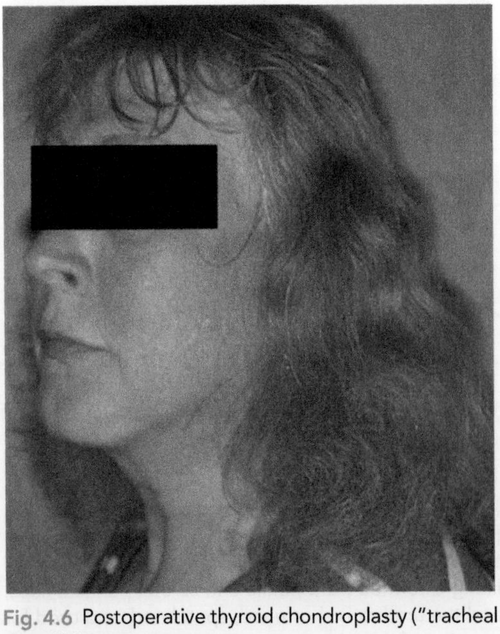

Preoperative Evaluation

The diagnosis of gender dysphoria is generally made by mental health providers, who then refer individuals for surgical evaluation. These professionals can come from a variety of backgrounds, including psychology, psychiatry, social work, mental health counseling, nursing, or medicine, and should have specific and ongoing training in evaluating and caring for transgender persons.[1] Before undergoing surgery, patients are

Fig. 4.6 Postoperative thyroid chondroplasty ("tracheal shave") in a transwoman.

BOX 4.2
Principles of chest surgery

The choice of technique depends on the volume of breast parenchyma, the degree of breast ptosis, the position and size of the nipple-areola complex, and the degree of skin elasticity.

Preoperative and postoperative photographs of double-incision mastectomy with free nipple-areola grafts. The procedure involved bilateral subcutaneous mastectomies, liposuction of chest, repositioning, and resizing of the nipple-areola complex.

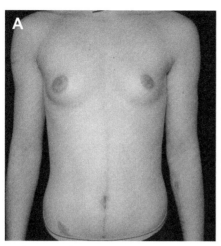
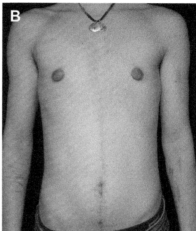

Fig. 4.7 Limited incision chest surgery in a transman. This patient has small, nonptotic breasts with good skin elasticity. The mastectomy was performed through an infra-areolar incision placed in a clockwise fashion from the 3 o'clock to 9 o'clock position. The nipples were reduced by a wedge resection, and the areolae were not resized.

evaluated to determine readiness and eligibility for genital reconstruction. Given the profound and usually irreversible nature of these procedures, the heterogeneity of the patient population, and the frequency of co-occurring medical and mental health issues, such assessments by trained mental health providers are essential for optimal care and correlate with positive outcomes.

If the surgeon is fortunate to work within a multidisciplinary team, the surgeon and mental health professional collaborate to ensure that the patient is adequately prepared before undergoing surgery. In this context, patients and providers benefit from the team's assistance with management of the perioperative and postoperative course.

The SOC necessitate one referral letter for chest or breast surgery, and 2 letters for genital surgery. Surgeons should have an understanding of what constitutes a thorough assessment, especially if they are not familiar with the referring provider.

A referral letter should provide, at a minimum, the following information:

- General identifying characteristics of the patient
- A description of the nature and duration of the therapist's relationship with the client
- A description of the onset, history, coping mechanisms, and severity of the gender dysphoria
- A statement describing and detailing the criteria that have been met
- A statement confirming the diagnosis of persistent, well-established gender dysphoria and a thorough assessment of any other diagnoses, past and present. If comorbid medical or mental health issues are present, the letter should state that these disorders are well-controlled
- The patient's rationale for surgery
- An indication that the referring mental health professional is willing to speak with the surgeon and coordinate care, if need be.

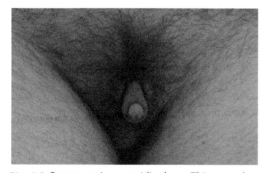

Fig. 4.8 Postoperative metoidioplasty. This procedure includes a scrotoplasty performed at the initial surgical setting, followed by subsequent placement of testicular implants and a mons resection. The metoidioplasty procedure does not create a phallus of sufficient size for placement of an erectile device. As such, the ability to engage in penetrative intercourse is limited.

BOX 4.3
Ideal phallic reconstruction

An aesthetic phallus with tactile and erogenous sensation, the ability to void while standing, an aesthetic scrotum, minimal morbidity, and the ability to experience sexual satisfaction.

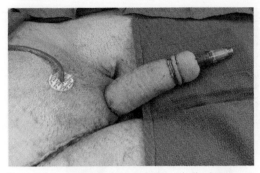

Fig. 4.9 Immediate postoperative phalloplasty performed with a radial forearm flap. This procedure includes urethral lengthening, glansplasty, and scrotoplasty.

For patients who are adequately screened and assessed, gender confirmation surgery greatly improves the individual's quality of life in virtually every area.

In addition to mental health evaluation, input from a patient's primary care doctor or endocrinologist is useful. Documentation of hormone therapy, if applicable, and confirmation that a patient is medically fit for surgery are important considerations. Tobacco use and obesity are relative contraindications for surgery. Tobacco can impair wound healing and result in flap failure. Patients should discontinue tobacco at least 6 weeks before surgery, and urine cotinine can be measured to assure patient compliance. Genital surgery can be difficult to perform in obese patients, and results may be compromised. In general, genital surgery should be performed on individuals with body mass indexes (BMIs) less than 30. For individuals with BMIs between 30 and 35, surgery can be considered based on body habitus and fat distribution. For BMIs greater than 35, weight loss should be encouraged before surgery. For some nongenital procedures (ie, chest or facial surgery), excess weight may not preclude surgery, but may be associated with higher rates of revision (Fig. 4.10).

For transwomen undergoing vaginoplasty, the physical examination should pay particular attention to the presence of inguinal hernia and/or pre-existing surgical incisions, including circumcision, which may affect either the vascular supply or the length of the penile flap.

For transmen undergoing metoidioplasty or phalloplasty, the physical examination should focus on the length of the virilized clitoris. For those individuals undergoing phalloplasty, particular attention should be paid to the pattern of hair growth at the donor site, which will be used for urethral reconstruction. In addition, an Allen test for those undergoing radial forearm phalloplasty should be performed to assess flow of the ulnar artery.

Before performing gender confirmation surgery, the surgeon must be satisfied that the diagnosis of gender dysphoria has been established. As noted by Dr J.J. Hage,[12] "the surgeon remains responsible for any diagnosis on the basis of which he (or she) performs surgical interventions." Direct communication between the surgeon and mental health professional(s) is recommended. This communication serves to educate the surgeon and to aid with his or her understanding of each patient's unique needs. It is also the responsibility of the surgeon to communicate pertinent operative findings as well as postoperative instructions with the health care team.[14]

Although multiple studies conducted at a variety of international centers confirm the efficacy of surgery and low complication rates,[15–20] the surgeon must be familiar with preoperative psychosocial risk factors that may increase the risk of postoperative complications. In a study investigating the standards and policies of 19 gender clinics in Europe and North America, a high degree of consistency regarding policies and criteria for approval of gender confirmation surgery was identified.[21] Based on questionnaire data, conditions that could result in delay or denial of surgery included psychosocial instability, married status, substance abuse, chronic or psychotic illness, and antisocial behavior. In addition, in a retrospective review of 136 patients who underwent gender confirmation surgery in Sweden, several preoperative factors were identified and reported to be associated with higher rates of unsatisfactory surgical outcomes. These factors included personal and social instability, unsuitable body build, and age older than 30 at the time of surgery. In addition, in this study, adequate family and social support were noted to be important for adequate postoperative functioning.[11]

Although understanding potential preoperative risk factors is important, their presence is not necessarily a contraindication to surgery. In a retrospective review of 232 transwomen, Lawrence[18] noted that no participants regretted gender confirmation surgery outright, and only 6% were occasionally regretful. In this study, dissatisfaction was associated with unsatisfactory surgical results, not other indicators of transgender typology, such as age at surgery, previous marriage or parenthood, or sexual orientation. This finding serves to reinforce the concept that the SOC are intended to provide flexible direction for the treatment of transgender persons. In addition, it must be emphasized that the SOC are not intended as barriers to surgery, but rather as a

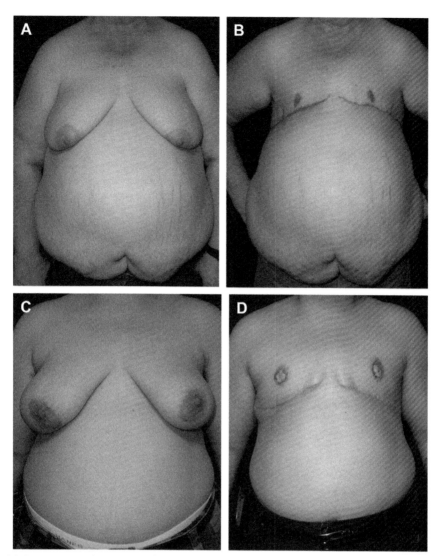

Fig. 4.10 (A) Preoperative photograph of morbidly obese patient undergoing chest surgery. (B) Postoperative result following chest surgery with double incision mastectomy and free nipple-areola grafts, liposuction of the chest, nipple and areola reduction, and areola repositioning. (C) Preoperative photograph of obese patient undergoing chest surgery. (D) Postoperative result following chest surgery with double-incision mastectomy and free nipple-areola grafts, liposuction of the chest, nipple, and areola reduction, and areola repositioning. Note hypopigmentation of the areola grafts and redundant tissue in the lateral and medial aspects of the chest incision.

means of identifying patients who may benefit from surgery.

Once the surgeon is satisfied that the diagnosis has been established, surgical therapy is considered. A preoperative surgical consultation is obtained, during which the procedure and postoperative course are described, the potential risks and benefits of surgery are reviewed, and the patient's questions are answered. Equally important is a discussion of the patient's expectations as well as an understanding of the limitations of surgery. In a follow-up study of 55 transgender patients

treated in Belgium, De Cuypere and colleagues[17] noted that the transgender person's expectations were met at an emotional and social level, but less so at the physical and sexual level; this occurred despite an indicated improvement in sex life and sexual excitement after gender confirmation surgery.[17] Based on these findings, it is recommended that discussion regarding sexual expectations be entertained before surgery.

If an individual decides to proceed with surgery, written documentation of informed consent should be included in the patient's chart.

REFERENCES

1. World Professional Association for Transgender Health Standards of Care. Available at: http://www.wpath.org/uploaded_files/140/files/Standards of Care, V7 Full Book.pdf. Accessed December 1, 2015.
2. Mate-Kole C, Freschi M, Robin A. A controlled study of psychological and social change after surgical gender reassignment in selected male transsexuals. Br J Psychiatry 1990;157:261–4.
3. Imbimbo C, Verze P, Palmieri A, et al. A report from a single institute's 14-year experience in treatment of male-to-female transsexuals. J Sex Med 2009; 6(10):2736–45.
4. Weyers S, Elaut E, De Sutter P, et al. Long-term assessment of the physical, mental, and sexual health among transsexual women. J Sex Med 2009;6(3):752–60.
5. Johansson A, Sundbom E, Hojerback T, et al. A five-year follow-up study of Swedish adults with gender identity disorder. Arch Sex Behav 2010; 39(6):1429–37.
6. Cohen-Kettenis P, Pfafflin F. Transgenderism and intersexuality in children and adolescence: making choices. Thousand Oaks (CA): Sage; 2003.
7. Meyer IH. Why lesbian, gay, bisexual, and transgender public health? Am J Public Health 2001; 91(6):856–9.
8. Cohen-Kettenis PT, Kuiper AJ. Transseksualiteit en psychotherapie. Tijdschr Psychoth 1984;3:153–66.
9. Seitz IA, Wu C, Retzlaff K, et al. Measurements and aesthetics of the mons pubis in normal weight females. Plast Reconstr Surg 2010;126(1):46e–8e.
10. Monstrey S, Hoebeke P, Selvaggi G, et al. Penile reconstruction: is the radial forearm flap really the standard technique? Plast Reconstr Surg 2009; 124(2):510–8.
11. Eldh J, Berg A, Gustafsson M. Long-term follow up after sex reassignment surgery. Scand J Plast Reconstr Surg Hand Surg 1997;31(1):39–45.
12. Hage JJ. Medical requirements and consequences of sex reassignment surgery. Med Sci L 1995;35(1): 17–24.
13. Edgerton MT. The role of surgery in the treatment of transsexualism. Ann Plast Surg 1984; 13(6):473–81.
14. Schechter LS. The surgeon's relationship with the physician prescribing hormones and the mental health professional: review for version 7 of the World Professional Association for Transgender Health's Standards of care. Int J Transgenderism 2009;11:222–5.
15. Monstrey S, Hoebeke P, Dhont M, et al. Surgical therapy in transsexual patients: a multi-disciplinary approach. Acta Chir Belg 2001;101(5):200–9.
16. Bowman C, Goldberg JM. Care of the patient undergoing sex reassignment surgery. Int J Transgenderism 2006;9(3–4):135–65.
17. De Cuypere G, T'Sjoen G, Beerten R, et al. Sexual and physical health after sex reassignment surgery. Arch Sex Behav 2005;34(6):679–90.
18. Lawrence A. Factors associated with satisfaction or regret following male-to-female sex reassignment surgery. Arch Sex Behav 2003;32(4):299–315.
19. Lobato M, Koff W, Manenti C, et al. Follow-up of sex reassignment surgery in transsexuals: a Brazilian cohort. Arch Sex Behav 2006;35:711–5.
20. Smith Y, Van Goozen S, Kuiper A, et al. Sex reassignment: outcomes and predictors of treatment for adolescent and adult transsexuals. Psychol Med 2005;35(1):89–99.
21. Petersen ME, Dickey R. Surgical sex reassignment: a comparative survey of international centers. Arch Sex Behav 1995;24(2):135–56.

CHAPTER 5

Surgical Therapy for Transwomen

Surgical conversion of the genitalia in transwomen has evolved since the use of skin grafts for creation of a neovagina in cases of vaginal agenesis.[1] The use of pedicled penile and scrotal flaps was described over 40 years ago, and despite technical refinements, remains the mainstay for neovaginal construction.[2–4] The vascular basis of these flaps is derived from 1 of 2 sources: (1) the femoral artery (deep and superficial external pudendal arteries) and (2) the internal pudendal artery (perineal branches, branches to the bulb and urethra of the penis, and the deep and dorsal penile branches) (Fig. 5.1).

Although a functional vaginoplasty is performed in a single stage, further feminization of the mons pubis can be performed at a second surgical stage. The labiaplasty, which can be performed under local anesthesia as an outpatient procedure 3 months after vaginoplasty, creates a convergent anterior labial commissure and provides additional clitoral hooding. However, with recent trends toward hair removal of the mons pubis, fewer individuals opt to proceed with secondary labiaplasty (Fig. 5.2).

The surgical options for vaginoplasty consist of 1 of 3 approaches: penile disassembly and inversion vaginoplasty, intestinal vaginoplasty, or nongenital flaps (Box 5.1). Most centers perform primary vaginoplasty with the penile disassembly and inversion vaginoplasty technique using an anteriorly based penile skin flap combined with a posteriorly based scrotal-perineal flap and/or skin graft. However, intestinal vaginoplasty, typically reserved for revision cases, is a first-line surgical therapy at some centers. The advantage of intestinal vaginoplasty is the creation of a vascularized 12- to 15-cm vagina with a moist lining, lessening the requirements for postoperative vaginal dilation as well as the need for lubrication during intercourse. However, the drawbacks of intestinal vaginoplasty include the need for an intra-abdominal operation with a bowel anastomosis and the potential for excess neovaginal secretions with a malodorous discharge. Because of their soft tissue bulk, nongenital flaps are typically considered for reconstruction following oncologic resections, traumatic repair, or reconstruction following infection. Alternatively, some individuals undergoing vaginoplasty for gender dysphoria do not contemplate vaginal intercourse. Sometimes referred to as a "zero-depth" procedure, this method is used to construct external genitalia (mons pubis, labia majora, labia minora and vestibular lining, and clitoris) without a vaginal canal.

Some individuals may undergo an orchiectomy as an independent procedure before vaginoplasty. Orchiectomy may assist with partial relief of dysphoria as well as reducing medication dosages. In such cases, an incision at the penoscrotal junction is preferred to an inguinal approach. The penoscrotal incision allows access to both the right and the left testicles and spermatic cords while preserving the vascular supply to the penile flap should later vaginoplasty be requested (Fig. 5.3).

Regardless of the technique used, hormones are discontinued approximately 2 weeks before surgery to reduce the risk of venous thromboembolism, and a preoperative bowel preparation is administered (Box 5.2). Before surgery, sequential compression devices (SCD) are placed, and intravenous antibiotics are administered. Following induction of general anesthesia, chemoprophylaxis for venous thromboembolism is administered subcutaneously (either fractionated or unfractionated heparin depending on institutional policies); the patient is positioned in lithotomy position; bony prominences are padded; the arms are abducted on foam rests with flexion at the elbows; an upper body forced-air surgical warming blanket is placed; and an indwelling urinary catheter is inserted under sterile conditions after the patient is prepared and draped (Fig. 5.4). The patient's position may vary when an intestinal vaginoplasty is performed robotically.

PENILE DISASSEMBLY AND INVERSION

Hair removal, whether by electrolysis or laser, is completed as thoroughly as possible from the penile shaft and central perineum and scrotum (Fig. 5.5) before penile inversion vaginoplasty. Preoperative depilation helps to

---

BOX 5.1
Surgical options for vaginoplasty

When vaginoplasty is performed for gender dysphoria, most centers use the penile disassembly and inversion vaginoplasty technique. In revision cases, or for primary cases with inadequate penile length, an intestinal vaginoplasty may be chosen. When vaginoplasty is performed for oncologic reconstruction, nongenital flaps are most often used.

Options

    Penile disassembly and inversion vaginoplasty

        Full-length scrotoperineal flap (± skin graft)

        Limited scrotoperineal flap (± skin graft)

    Intestinal vaginoplasty

    Nongenital flaps

Considerations

    Indication

        Gender dysphoria

        Oncologic, traumatic, infectious

    Patient goals

        Vaginal intercourse

        "Zero depth"

    Penile length

    (±) Circumcision

    Primary versus revision

---

prevent intravaginal hair growth. Adequate hair removal can take 3 to 6 months to complete and should not be performed within 2 weeks of surgery.

Primary vaginoplasty surgery most commonly involves penile disassembly and inversion with an anteriorly based penile flap. Although a variety of technical modifications are described in the

---

BOX 5.2
Bowel preparation regimen

The same bowel preparation is used for vaginoplasty, metoidioplasty, and phalloplasty procedures. Ingredients are available over the counter:

- Magnesium citrate (10 oz.)
- MiraLAX 238 g
- Can of 7-Up or Diet 7-Up
- Gatorade (if diabetic, Propel Fitness Water)

The day before surgery, you must have a clear liquid diet (apple juice, soda, Jell-O, chicken broth, and tea) for the entire day. Red dye–colored products should be avoided.

At 11 AM, drink a full bottle of magnesium citrate mixed equally with 7-Up or Diet 7-Up; drink this within 15 minutes.

For lunch, continue on a clear liquid diet.

At 3 PM, mix MiraLAX 238 g with Gatorade (or Propel) 64 oz. and drink within 2 hours.

For dinner, continue on a clear liquid diet.

Do not drink any liquids containing red dye.

Nothing to eat or drink after midnight.

literature, the penile disassembly and inversion technique uses the penile skin and a second, posteriorly based, scrotal-perineal flap to construct the vaginal cavity (Fig. 5.6).[5] The author's preferred technique is described herein: the labia majora are formed from the lateral aspects of the scrotum; the neoclitoris is formed from the dorsal glans penis; and the labia minora and vestibular lining are formed with the creation of a urethral flap inset within the penile flap. The penile urethra is shortened, spatulated, and everted to create the urethra, urethral meatus, and portions of the labia minora and vestibular lining (Fig. 5.7). Depending on the length of the penis and previous surgical history (ie, circumcision), skin grafts may be required for additional vaginal depth. Full-thickness skin grafts may be harvested from discarded portions of the scrotum. If this is insufficient, additional full-thickness skin grafts may be harvested with a Pfannenstiel incision.[6] Alternatively, split-thickness skin grafts may be harvested from the lower abdomen or mons region. However, the donor site of the split-thickness skin grafts may be left with areas of hypopigmentation depending on the depth of harvest and the patient's skin tone.

The procedure is begun with the creation of a posteriorly based scrotal-perineal flap. The dimensions of this flap may vary, depending on whether the scrotal-perineal flap forms the entire posterior vaginal wall or, alternatively, is inset into the penile flap. For individuals who are not circumcised, a smaller, limited scrotal-perineal flap is typically chosen. If used to form the entire posterior vaginal wall, the flap typically measures approximately 15 cm in length, has a base diameter of 3 to 4 cm, and is approximately 6 to 8 cm in the largest transverse dimension. The flap needs to be of sufficient width so as not to limit the vaginal introitus. However, the borders of the flap are maintained within the boundaries of the scrotum to create a smooth, graded, and contiguous appearance to the newly formed labia majora. In addition, the lateral aspect of the flap is designed in a "V-shaped" fashion so as not to create a circular introitus, thereby minimizing the chance of introital contracture. The flap is centered cephalad to the anus and elevated in an extrasphincteric plane, with care taken not to injure the external anal sphincter (Fig. 5.8). The flap should be thin, and its base is elevated so as to maintain a broad subcutaneous pedicle without creating a rectangular appearance to the posterior labial commissure (Fig. 5.9).

Following elevation of the scrotoperineal flap, the penile flap is developed with an incision on the ventral aspect of the phallus, located along the midline raphe (Fig. 5.10). The length of the incision along the ventral penis depends on the length of the phallus, and whether the individual has been circumcised. If there is sufficient penile skin, the incision ends approximately halfway along the ventral phallus. This incision design will leave the distal penile flap tubularized. In such instances, the limited scrotoperineal flap is inset into the tubularized penile flap.

Following elevation of both the penile and the scrotoperineal flaps, access to the testicles and spermatic cords is established, allowing the performance of bilateral orchiectomies. The orchiectomies, including resection of the spermatic cords, are carried out at the level of the external inguinal ring (Figs. 5.11 and 5.12). Resection of the spermatic cord at this level allows the spermatic cord to retract within the inguinal canal and prevents a palpable bulge in the groin area. The skin of the penile shaft is then circumferentially incised at the junction of the glans and penile shaft, facilitating elevation of the penile flap (Fig. 5.13). This facilitates separation of the penile skin from the underlying corpora cavernosa and corpora spongiosum, as well as the underlying muscles, the ischiocavernosus and bulbospongiosus muscles, respectively (Fig. 5.14).

The vaginal cavity is developed by dissection between the prostate and rectum (Fig. 5.15). During this dissection, injury to the rectum may occur. Dissection follows Denonvilliers fascia until the peritoneal reflection is reached. Most of the dissection is performed bluntly; however, release of the attachments between the prostate and rectum may require sharp division. The levator ani muscles are incised with electrocautery to allow further lateral expansion of the neovaginal cavity (Fig. 5.16). Adequate dissection of the neovaginal space is essential in creating and maintaining adequate vaginal depth and width. Once the vaginal cavity is created, the superficial perineal muscles are resected. Resection of the bulbospongiosus and ischiocavernosus muscles aids with expansion of the introitus and exposure of the underlying corpora spongiosum and corpora cavernosa (Fig. 5.17). At this point, the corpora spongiosum is separated from the corpora cavernosa (Fig. 5.18). In order to further open the vaginal cavity, the corpora spongiosum is resected and oversewn at the level of the urethral bulb (Fig. 5.19). If excess erectile tissue is not removed, this tissue may become engorged during sexual arousal and restrict entry into the vaginal cavity.[7]

The neoclitoris is then fashioned from the dorsal glans penis and elevated with the dorsal neurovascular bundle. The dissection of the neurovascular pedicle is performed deep to Buck fascia, along the dorsal surface of the corpora cavernosa.[8] Dissection of the neurovascular pedicle continues proximally, to the pubic symphysis, thereby exposing the divergence of the underlying corpora cavernosa (Fig. 5.20). The corpora cavernosa are resected at the pubis, leaving a short remnant of the corpora on either side. The retained corpora will be oversewn and sutured approximately to form a base upon which the neoclitoris will be positioned (S. Monstrey, personal communication, 2003) (Fig. 5.21A). The pedicle of the neoclitoris is sutured to the fascia of the anterior abdominal wall, and the neoclitoris is sutured to the underlying corporal base (Fig. 5.21B, C).

In order to aid with positioning of the penile flap, the skin of the mons and lower abdomen may be elevated to the umbilicus and advanced inferiorly. The advancement flap is then suture stabilized to the anterior abdominal wall (Fig. 5.22). In some individuals, this advancement flap facilitates intravaginal positioning of the penile flap.[9] Depending on the length of the penile flap, skin grafts may be required to increase vaginal depth. These skin grafts may be harvested as full-thickness grafts from the unused portions of the scrotum, from the groin crease, or from the lower abdomen (see Fig. 5.8C). In addition, split-thickness skin grafts may be harvested from the mons or lower abdominal region.[10] The skin-lined neovaginal cavity is then created by suturing the scrotal-perineal flap to the penile flap, and the tubularized construct is positioned intravaginally (Fig. 5.23). Fibrin sealant may be used to aid with hemostasis and adherence of the tubularized flaps to the dissected vaginal cavity. Drains are placed on either side of the vaginal cavity.

For insetting of the clitoris and urethra, a "Y"-shaped incision is made in the penile flap (Fig. 5.24). The penile urethra is transferred through this incision (Fig. 5.25), shortened, and incised ventrally. This urethral flap, through which the glans penis (neoclitoris) will be placed, aids in the formation of the labia minora and vestibular lining and provides clitoral hooding and a prepuce to the neoclitoris (Fig. 5.26). Sufficient length should be created between the urethral meatus and clitoris to simulate the vestibular lining of the natal female.

The scrotal skin is then tailored to form the labia majora, and the incisions are closed in a layered fashion with absorbable sutures. A silastic stent is placed within the vaginal cavity, and dressings are applied (Fig. 5.27).

Although most surgeons perform a single-stage vaginoplasty, an optional second stage, referred to as a labiaplasty, may be performed approximately 3 months after vaginoplasty for further feminization of the mons pubis. The labiaplasty involves a local tissue rearrangement, frequently in the form of multiple "z"-plasties, in order to create convergence of the labia majora and provide additional clitoral hooding (Fig. 5.28).

Technical variations in the performance of vaginoplasty include the use of a urethral flap inset within the penile skin designed to lengthen, widen, or provide lubrication to the vaginal cavity.[11] In addition, intravaginal placement of the glans penis to act as a neocervix has been described.[12]

The postoperative care consists of a variable period of bed rest, typically 4 to 5 days, during which a silastic stent is used to maintain the vaginal cavity. A urinary catheter remains in place until the vaginal packing is removed and ambulation is initiated, typically 5 to 6 days after surgery. Both mechanical and chemoprophylaxis for venous thromboembolism are used, and hormonal therapy is reinitiated once the patient is ambulatory (Box 5.3).

On removal of the vaginal stent, a regimen of vaginal dilation with a prosthesis is begun (Box 5.4). Initially, dilation of the neovaginal cavity is performed 3 to 4 times daily for 6 weeks. The frequency of dilation is reduced over a period of 2 to 3 months, ultimately requiring dilation 2 to 3 times per week (Fig. 5.29). This schedule may vary depending on the frequency of vaginal intercourse. In addition, intermittent vaginal douching with a dilute soap solution is performed in order to remove intravaginal debris. This vaginal douching is initially performed 2 to 3 times per week beginning 3 to 4 weeks after surgery (Box 5.5).

INTESTINAL VAGINOPLASTY

In cases of congenital vaginal agenesis, insufficient penile length, or the event that vaginal depth following penile inversion vaginoplasty is inadequate, vaginoplasty typically requires either skin grafting, local and/or regional nongenital flaps, or intestinal transposition. Although a skin graft placed through a perineal approach may alleviate the need for an intra-abdominal procedure, the secondary dissection of the previously operated on vaginal cavity may be difficult because of scarring and limited visualization. In addition, donor sites for full-thickness skin grafts may be unavailable, and hypopigmentation from split-thickness skin graft donor sites may be undesirable. Furthermore, skin grafts require regular postoperative dilation in order to prevent contraction of the neovagina. Local and regional

BOX 5.3
Postoperative orders: vaginoplasty

The patient is transferred directly to the hospital bed from the operating room table.

Admit to Dr Schechter

Status postvaginoplasty

Stable

Vitals: Every 4 hours

Allergies:

Activity: Strict bed rest for 5 days (until vaginal packing removed by Dr Schechter)

May ambulate and shower with assistance after packing removed by Dr Schechter on postoperative day 5

Dilation to begin after vaginal packing removed on postoperative day 5

Nursing: Input/Output, drains × 2 to bulb suction, spirometry 10×/h, urinary catheter to gravity drainage (remove urinary catheter on postoperative day 5 after vaginal packing removed by Dr Schechter), SCDs at all times

Diet: Nothing by mouth except ice chips after surgery, may advance to clear liquids if tolerating ice chips

Intravenous fluids: lactated Ringer solution at 150 mL/h, change to dextrose 5% 0.45 normal saline with 20 meq KCl postoperative day 1

Medication:

Cefazolin 1 g intravenously piggyback every 8 h × 3 doses, then discontinue

Patient-controlled analgesia (PCA) as ordered (morphine 1 mg 12 min, may substitute with dilaudid)

Acetaminophen/hydrocodone 10 mg orally every 4 to 6 h as necessary when PCA discontinued

Metoclopramide 10 mg intravenously every 6 h (may use Zofran)

Zolpidem 1 mg orally every bedtime as necessary, begin postoperative day 1

Docusate sodium 100 mg orally twice a day when taking regular diet

Enoxaparin 40 mg subcutaneously every day starting postoperative day 1 after seen by Dr Schechter

Laboratory tests: complete blood count (CBC) in recovery room, CBC and electrolytes postoperative days 1 and 2

Dressing supplies:

Surgilube at bedside

Gauze pads at bedside

Abdominal pads at bedside

4″ foam tape at bedside

Suture removal kit at bedside

Surgicel at bedside

Wash cloths and chux pads at bedside

---

nongenital flaps include the use of various thigh or perineal-based flaps. The advantages of these nongenital flaps include less risk of postoperative contraction. However, many of these flaps are bulky, limit the size of the neovagina, and provide no intrinsic lubrication.

The advantage of intestinal transposition, especially in revision cases, is the provision of a reliable length of vascularized tissue capable of mucus production and the provision of lubrication for vaginal intercourse. Intestinal transposition may use either the small or the large intestine; however, the sigmoid colon is the most commonly used. The advantage of the sigmoid colon is the larger luminal diameter and less copious secretions as compared with that of the jejunum or ileum. Before performing the sigmoid vaginoplasty, a preoperative colonoscopy is performed so as to evaluate for pre-existing colorectal malignancies. As with penile disassembly and inversion vaginoplasty, a bowel preparation is prescribed the day before surgery.

> **BOX 5.4**
> **Postoperative vaginal dilation instructions**
>
> Vaginal dilation will begin when your vaginal packing is removed. This will occur on the fourth to sixth day after surgery, and the dilators will be provided to you before discharge. Dr Schechter will review specific instructions regarding dilation.
>
> 1. Begin with the smallest dilator lubricated with KY Jelly. Gently insert the dilator the entire length of the vagina and allow the dilator to remain in place for 5 to 10 minutes. One dilation each day should include the use of bacitracin antibiotic ointment. Bacitracin should be used for the first 6 weeks after surgery.
>
> 2. When inserting and rotating the first dilator becomes easy, progress to the next size. This process should take about 2 to 4 weeks.
>
> 3. Dilation should be performed 3 to 4 times daily for the first 6 weeks after surgery. After 6 weeks, the dilation should be performed twice daily for 3 months and then daily for the next 2 months. Six months after surgery, dilation should be performed 2 to 3 times each week. If you notice the dilation becoming more difficult, you should increase the frequency.
>
> 4. The dilators should be thoroughly cleansed after each use with an antibacterial soap.
>
> Dilator care:
>
> 1. Soak the dilator in a betadine solution for no more than 10 to 15 minutes before use
>
> 2. Wash the dilator with an antibacterial hand soap after each use

The sigmoid vaginoplasty is performed in conjunction with general surgery. The patient is placed in the lithotomy position, and a combined abdominal and perineal approach is used. The lithotomy position permits visualization and protection of the bladder and urethra anteriorly and the rectum posteriorly. The general surgery team harvests the sigmoid colon while, concurrently, the plastic surgery team performs the perineal dissection. Recently, the sigmoid harvest has been performed using a combination of robotic and laparoscopic techniques. Traditionally, the inferior mesenteric artery and vein provide the vascular supply of the intestinal flap. More recently, the inferior mesenteric pedicle is divided at its origin from the aorta, and the vascular basis of the flap is antegrade flow through the marginal artery. A secondary blood supply to the mobilized intestinal segment derives from the superior hemorrhoidal artery, receiving retrograde flow through the ascending branch of the left colic artery. This principle is a similar construct used for coloanal reconstruction following resection of a low rectal cancer. However, in cases of intestinal vaginoplasty, during transection of the bowel, the marginal artery to the neovaginal intestinal segment must be maintained.

The author's preferred technique is described herein: The plastic surgery team begins the perineal dissection with release of the constricted vaginal introitus, thereby exposing the perineal cavity (Fig. 5.30). Concurrent with the pelvic dissection, the general surgery team begins the abdominal portion of the

> **BOX 5.5**
> **Postoperative vaginal douching instructions**
>
> Typically performed in the shower:
>
> 1. Place a few drops of an antibacterial liquid soap in the douche bag and fill with warm water.
>
> 2. Insert the tip of the douche a few inches into the vagina and gently squeeze the bag.
>
> 3. Repeat this process with clear water to remove the soap residue.
>
> 4. This should be performed 2 to 3 times per week, beginning 2 weeks after discharge from the hospital.
>
> 5. After 6 weeks, douching should be performed 1 to 2 times each week.
>
> A yellowish-brown discharge may be noted for the first few weeks after surgery. In addition, you may notice sutures and debris in the discharge.

procedure. Standard laparoscopy is used to mobilize the left colon, including division of the inferior mesenteric artery and vein at their origins. The left colon, including the splenic flexure, is completely mobilized (Fig. 5.31A). At this point, the laparoscopic portion of the procedure is concluded, and the robot is docked (Fig. 5.31B). The use of the robot facilitates anterior mesorectal mobilization. This dissection allows complete exposure of Denonvilliers fascia with preservation of the pelvic plexus and middle rectal arteries. The levator ani muscles are incised laterally in order to widen the vaginal cavity, and the abdominal and perineal dissections are communicated. Sufficient space is created between the abdominal and perineal dissections so as not to compress the vascular pedicle of the transferred sigmoid colon.

With preservation of the marginal artery, the mobilized colon is transected at the upper rectum (Fig. 5.32). A 12- to 15-cm segment of sigmoid colon (Fig. 5.33) is transferred in an isoperistaltic fashion, and the defunctionalized sigmoid colon is interposed between the urethra and bladder, anteriorly, and the rectum, posteriorly (Fig. 5.34). The mesentery of the defunctionalized sigmoid colon may be sewn to the pelvic brim, if necessary, to prevent torsion of the vascular pedicle. If mobilization of the left colon is limited, the sigmoid segment may be inset in a retroperistaltic fashion. In addition, if the mesentery of the distal sigmoid colon is bulky and limits mobilization, the distal half of the sigmoid may be resected, preserving the superior hemorrhoidal artery. Preserving the superior hemorrhoidal artery may facilitate passage of the more proximal sigmoid colon into the perineum.

An end-to-end colonic anastomosis is performed to restore intestinal continuity (Fig. 5.35A). The distal stump of the defunctionalized sigmoid colon (neovagina) is separated from the colorectal anastomosis so as to reduce the risk of fistulization. An omental flap may be interposed between these suture lines (Fig. 5.35B).

The distal portion of the defunctionalized sigmoid colon forms the neovaginal introitus (Fig. 5.36). The colon is sutured to the perineal skin with a single layer of absorbable sutures (Fig. 5.37). In order to prevent contraction of the introitus, the colon is inset obliquely at the perineal skin surface (Fig. 5.38).

The neovagina is packed for 2 to 3 days, and a urinary catheter is maintained during this time. Intravenous antibiotics are discontinued after 24 hours, and mechanical and chemoprophylaxis for venous thromboembolism are used. Upon return of bowel function and oral intake, the patient is discharged from the hospital. Hormone therapy is resumed once the patient is ambulatory. Dilation of the introitus is required; however, deep vaginal dilation is not necessary.

The potential drawback of intestinal-based flaps includes secretions, most notably with the small intestine, and possible malodorous discharge with the large intestine. Additional concerns include the possibility of diversion colitis in the defunctionalized sigmoid colon, and, because the colonic mucosa may be somewhat friable, small amounts of postcoital bleeding may occur. Finally, annual speculum examination of the sigmoid vaginoplasty is recommended because of the risk of gastrointestinal malignancies in the sigmoid vagina.

COMPLICATIONS

Early postoperative complications from penile disassembly and inversion vaginoplasty or intestinal vaginoplasty include bleeding, infection, and delayed wound healing. Additional early or late complications include rectovaginal fistula, urinary stream abnormalities, inadequate vaginal depth or a constricted introitus, partial flap loss, loss of neoclitoral sensation, inability to orgasm, and an unsatisfactory cosmetic appearance. There is also the possibility of stenosis of the neovagina, requiring a secondary revision.

In the event of a rectal injury, the rectum is closed in a layered fashion. Should a rectovaginal fistula develop, there may be a need for fecal diversion with either a colostomy or an ileostomy.

Although minor urinary stream abnormalities are not uncommon, the risk of stenosis of the neourethral meatus may be reduced by spatulation of the urethra.

It is also imperative that the individual continue routine dilation after penile disassembly and inversion vaginoplasty so as to reduce the likelihood of vaginal stenosis. Although the frequency of dilation may be reduced with sexual intercourse, pedicled penile flaps and skin grafts still require compliance with vaginal dilation.

AFTER-DISCHARGE CARE

Postoperatively, patients are encouraged to wear dark, loose fitting clothing and avoid tight elastic straps at the groin region. A pad placed in the underwear is often required for several weeks following surgery. Although ambulation is encouraged, time spent sitting should be minimized so as to reduce perineal swelling. Patients are encouraged to elevate their legs as much as possible to aid with reduction of perineal edema.

Individuals who travel should minimize their luggage, because lifting requirements are limited to less than 15 pounds for the first several weeks after surgery. In addition, it is recommended that patients stay in the area for several days after surgery before returning home.

For the first 6 weeks after surgery, activity is limited; patients should not lift more than 15 pounds or engage in strenuous exercise or vaginal intercourse. Six weeks after surgery, usual activities can be resumed, including exercise and vaginal intercourse.

ADDITIONAL PROCEDURES FOR TRANSWOMEN

Additional procedures for transwomen include breast augmentation, facial feminization, thyroid chondroplasty ("tracheal shave"), and body contouring. The goal of these procedures is to remove the secondary sexual characteristics and stigmata associated with the biological male appearance. The timing of these surgeries in relation to genital surgery may vary between centers as well as within individual centers. It is not uncommon for feminizing procedures to be performed before genital surgery so as to improve the individual's sense of well-being.[13] As with genital surgery, hormone therapy is discontinued 2 weeks before surgery, and SCDs are placed. For high-risk individuals, chemoprophylaxis for venous thromboembolism is administered subcutaneously (either fractionated or unfractionated heparin depending on institutional policies), unless the patient is undergoing eyelid surgery.

Breast Augmentation

Following hormonal therapy, there is frequently some breast growth in the transwoman. However, the degree of breast growth is often inadequate, and individuals continue to wear external prostheses or padded bras. As such, augmentation mammaplasty may be requested. Anatomic differences between the male and female chest are relevant as to implant selection, incision choice, and pocket location.[14]

The natal male chest is not only wider than the natal female chest, but the pectoralis major muscle is usually more developed. Furthermore, the natal male areola is smaller than the natal female areola; the distance between the nipple and inframammary crease is less, and there is less ptosis in the natal male breast, even after hormonal therapy (Fig. 5.39).[15]

Although the principles of augmentation mammaplasty are similar to that of natal females, the broader chest, larger pectoralis muscle, and shorter distance between the nipple and inframammary crease warrant additional consideration. These anatomic characteristics may require lowering the inframammary crease and releasing the lower sternal attachments of the pectoralis major muscle (Fig. 5.40). When releasing the sternal attachments of the pectoralis muscle, the overlying pectoralis fascia is left intact. These maneuvers may assist with implant positioning relative to the position of the nipple areola complex and also help to prevent lateral implant displacement. Because of the wider chest wall diameter in natal males, a wide interbreast width is common, even with the selection of larger implants.

The implants may be placed in either a subglandular or a subpectoral pocket. This decision depends on the degree of breast growth in response to hormonal therapy. Subglandular implants may be more palpable and may have higher rates of capsular contracture due to less soft tissue coverage overlying the implant. However, subpectoral implants may be more prone to displacement due to the activity of the pectoralis major muscle. Nonetheless, the subpectoral position remains the most common pocket location.

In terms of incisions, transaxillary, periareolar, or inframammary crease approaches may be used and are tailored to the requests and the anatomy of the individual. Because of the smaller size of the natal male areola, and the frequent choice of large implant, an inframammary crease approach is most commonly chosen. Furthermore, with the increased use of form-stable implants, larger incisions are often required, also favoring an inframammary crease approach (Fig. 5.41).

Facial Feminization

Facial features may also be typically male or female. As such, surgery to "feminize" the face of transwomen is frequently requested. A variety of characteristics have been identified as male and are often associated with the forehead, nose, malar region, mandible, and thyroid cartilage. These differences include more pronounced supraorbital bossing in the natal male and a more continuous forehead curvature in the natal female.[16] The malar region is also more prominent in the natal female, and the natal female nose tends to be smaller, with a less acute glabellar angle than the natal male.[16,17] In addition, qualitative and quantitative differences in the skin, subcutaneous tissue, and hair also exist (Fig. 5.42).[18]

Because the natal female eyebrow is located above the supraorbital rim and has a more arched appearance than the natal male, typical procedures for facial feminization include a brow lift with advancement of the frontal hairline and frontal bone reduction. Although the brow lift may be performed with endoscopic techniques, reduction of the frontal bone and lateral brow is facilitated with the open approach. In addition, the open approach, performed through an anterior hairline incision, allows advancement of the frontal hairline, if desired. Before proceeding with reduction of the frontal bone, lateral skull films or a computed tomographic scan are obtained in order to assess the thickness of the anterior table of the frontal sinus. Depending on the thickness of the anterior table in relation to the degree of frontal bossing, craniofacial techniques may be used for the desired correction.

A feminizing rhinoplasty typically involves dorsal hump reduction, cephalic trim, elevation of the nasal tip, and osteotomies to narrow the nasal pyramid (Fig. 5.43). The chin and mandible represent additional anatomic sites that individuals may want to feminize. Based on the individual's anatomy, either chin implants or osteoplastic genioplasty may be required. In addition, reduction of the masseter muscle or contouring of the mandibular angle may be performed through intraoral incisions. Other procedures, such as upper lip shortening, facelift, blepharoplasty, malar implants, hair transplantation, injectable fillers, and skin resurfacing, may also be requested (Figs. 5.44 and 5.45).

Thyroid Chondroplasty

Reduction thyroid chondroplasty is often requested to reduce the appearance of the "Adam's apple" or prominent thyroid cartilage (pomus Adamus) (Fig. 5.46). The procedure is typically performed as an outpatient under general or local anesthesia with sedation. The procedure is performed through a transverse incision in a naturally occurring skin crease. Following vertical division of the middle cervical fascia, the sternothyroid and thyrohyoid muscles are retracted laterally. The perichondrium is incised, and a subperichondrial dissection is performed with care so as not to enter the thyrohyoid membrane. On the posterior surface of the cartilage, subperichondrial dissection is performed inferiorly to the thyroepiglottic ligament. Dissection stops at this point so as not to injure the insertion of the vocal cords or destabilize the epiglottis. Identification of the insertion of the vocal cords may be facilitated with fiberoptic laryngoscopy performed through a laryngeal mask airway (LMA) by the anesthesiologist.[19] Resection of the thyroid cartilage is performed between the superior thyroid notch in the midline and the superior thyroid tubercle superolaterally (Fig. 5.47). The perichondrium is reapproximated, and the incision is closed in a layered fashion (Fig. 5.48).[20]

Body Contouring

Body contouring procedures such as abdominoplasty, liposuction, and lipofilling of the hips and buttocks may be requested to feminize one's silhouette. As a result of puberty and estrogen, natal females have wider hips and increased fat distribution in the buttocks, thighs, and hips as compared with natal males. Similarly, testosterone tends to reduce the amount of body fat in natal males, who tend to carry fat in their waist and abdomen.

Body contouring procedures follow similar principles as those in the natal female and are not typically performed at the same surgical setting as vaginoplasty (Fig. 5.49).

Voice Surgery

Because hormonal intervention does not typically affect vocal pitch, a deep voice may represent a residual stigma of masculinity. Some individuals may find vocal therapy useful. In addition, various techniques to shorten the vocal cords, increase vocal cord tension, or reduce vibrating vocal cord mass may be performed to raise vocal pitch.[21] However, the efficacy of such surgery is debated.[22,23]

A

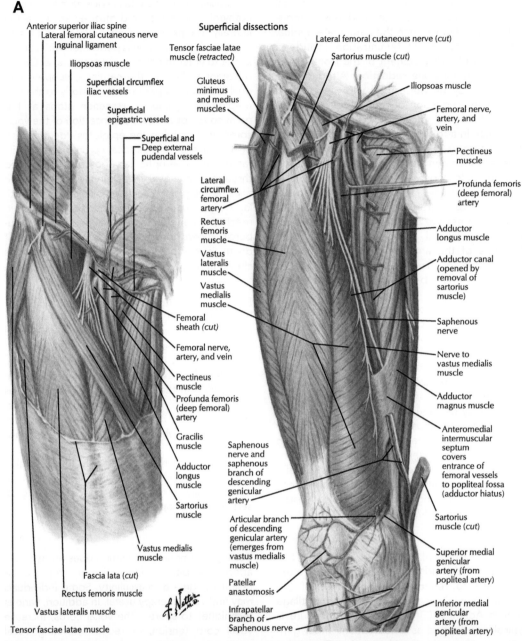

Superficial dissections

Anterior superior iliac spine
Lateral femoral cutaneous nerve
Inguinal ligament
Tensor fasciae latae muscle (retracted)
Iliopsoas muscle
Lateral femoral cutaneous nerve (cut)
Sartorius muscle (cut)
Superficial circumflex iliac vessels
Gluteus minimus and medius muscles
Iliopsoas muscle
Superficial epigastric vessels
Femoral nerve, artery, and vein
Superficial and Deep external pudendal vessels
Pectineus muscle
Lateral circumflex femoral artery
Profunda femoris (deep femoral) artery
Rectus femoris muscle
Adductor longus muscle
Vastus lateralis muscle
Adductor canal (opened by removal of sartorius muscle)
Vastus medialis muscle
Saphenous nerve
Femoral sheath (cut)
Nerve to vastus medialis muscle
Femoral nerve, artery, and vein
Pectineus muscle
Adductor magnus muscle
Profunda femoris (deep femoral) artery
Anteromedial intermuscular septum covers entrance of femoral vessels to popliteal fossa (adductor hiatus)
Gracilis muscle
Saphenous nerve and saphenous branch of descending genicular artery
Adductor longus muscle
Sartorius muscle
Sartorius muscle (cut)
Articular branch of descending genicular artery (emerges from vastus medialis muscle)
Superior medial genicular artery (from popliteal artery)
Vastus medialis muscle
Patellar anastomosis
Fascia lata (cut)
Rectus femoris muscle
Inferior medial genicular artery (from popliteal artery)
Vastus lateralis muscle
Infrapatellar branch of Saphenous nerve
Tensor fasciae latae muscle

f. Netter

Fig. 5.1 (A) Anatomy of the superficial femoral artery and femoral vein. The relevant branches include the external pudendal vessels, the superficial inferior epigastric vessels, the superficial circumflex iliac vessels, and the great saphenous vein. (B) Anatomy of the internal pudendal artery and vein and its branches. (Copyright © 2016. Used with permission of Elsevier. All rights reserved. www.netterimages.com.)

B

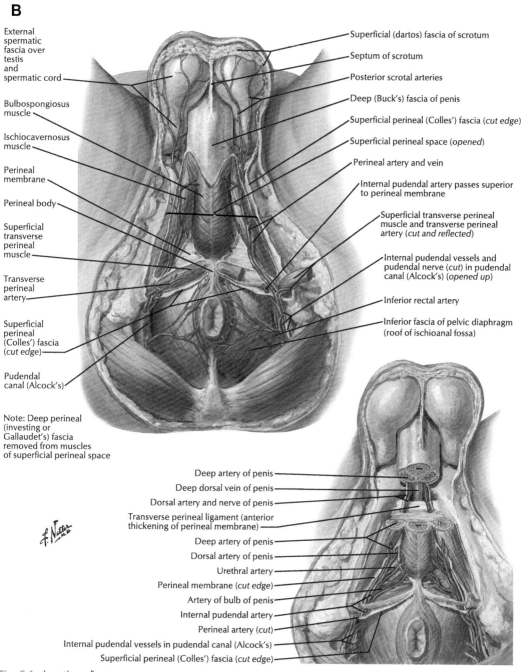

External spermatic fascia over testis and spermatic cord

Bulbospongiosus muscle

Ischiocavernosus muscle

Perineal membrane

Perineal body

Superficial transverse perineal muscle

Transverse perineal artery

Superficial perineal (Colles') fascia (cut edge)

Pudendal canal (Alcock's)

Note: Deep perineal (investing or Gallaudet's) fascia removed from muscles of superficial perineal space

Superficial (dartos) fascia of scrotum

Septum of scrotum

Posterior scrotal arteries

Deep (Buck's) fascia of penis

Superficial perineal (Colles') fascia (cut edge)

Superficial perineal space (opened)

Perineal artery and vein

Internal pudendal artery passes superior to perineal membrane

Superficial transverse perineal muscle and transverse perineal artery (cut and reflected)

Internal pudendal vessels and pudendal nerve (cut) in pudendal canal (Alcock's) (opened up)

Inferior rectal artery

Inferior fascia of pelvic diaphragm (roof of ischioanal fossa)

Deep artery of penis

Deep dorsal vein of penis

Dorsal artery and nerve of penis

Transverse perineal ligament (anterior thickening of perineal membrane)

Deep artery of penis

Dorsal artery of penis

Urethral artery

Perineal membrane (cut edge)

Artery of bulb of penis

Internal pudendal artery

Perineal artery (cut)

Internal pudendal vessels in pudendal canal (Alcock's)

Superficial perineal (Colles') fascia (cut edge)

Fig. 5.1   (continued)

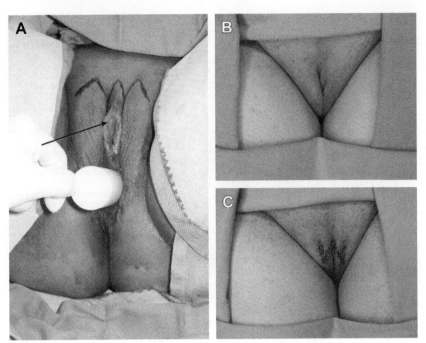

Fig. 5.2 (A) Postoperative vaginoplasty with penile disassembly and inversion technique. The arrow indicates the urethral flap inset within the penile flap, helping to form the labia minora and clitoral hood. Preoperative markings for secondary labiaplasty (dilator in place demonstrating neovaginal depth). (B) Postoperative vaginoplasty, before labiaplasty. (C) Postoperative labiaplasty performed to provide additional convergence of anterior labial commissure.

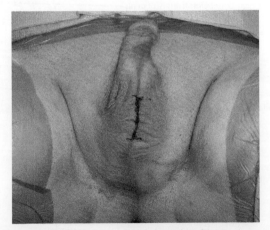

Fig. 5.3 Preferred incision, at penoscrotal junction, when bilateral orchiectomies are performed without vaginoplasty. An incision at the penoscrotal junction maintains the ability to perform a vaginoplasty using a scrotoperineal flap, and it also preserves the blood supply to the subsequent penile flap. An inguinal incision may divide the blood supply to the penile flap (pudendal vessels) should a vaginoplasty be requested at a later date.

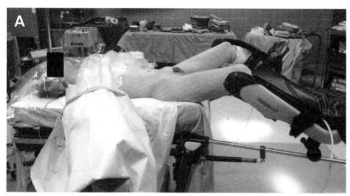

Fig. 5.4 Lithotomy position. SCD boots are placed; the arms are abducted on foam rests with flexion at the elbows, and an upper body forced-air surgical warming blanket is placed.

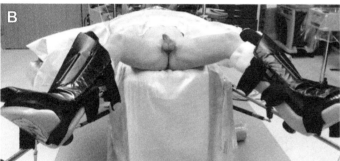

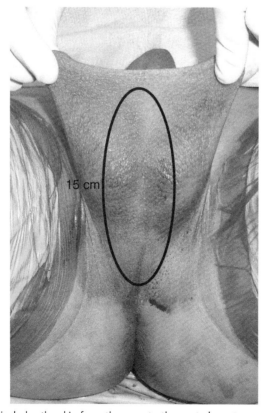

Fig. 5.5 Area of depilation includes the skin from the anus to the central scrotum as well as the penile shaft. The marked area corresponds to the approximate dimensions of the scrotoperineal flap. This tissue will form the posterior vaginal wall.

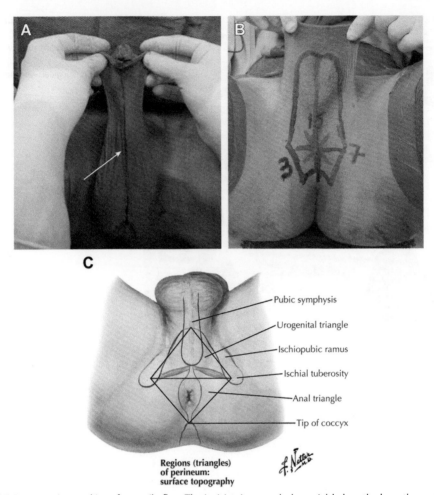

Regions (triangles) of perineum: surface topography

Pubic symphysis
Urogenital triangle
Ischiopubic ramus
Ischial tuberosity
Anal triangle
Tip of coccyx

Fig. 5.6 (*A*) Preoperative markings for penile flap. The incision is extended a variable length along the ventral penile shaft (*white arrow*). (*B*) Preoperative markings for scroto-perineal flap, when the flap is used to form the entire posterior vaginal wall. The asterisk indicates the position of the central tendon. This is the location at which the vaginal introitus will be located. (*C*) The insert demonstrates the position of the urogenital and anal triangles in relation to the scroto-perineal flap. ([*C*] Copyright © 2016. Used with permission of Elsevier. All rights reserved. www.netterimages.com.)

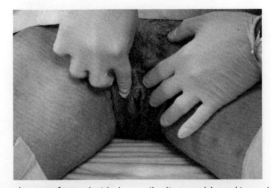

Fig. 5.7 Postoperative vaginoplasty performed with the penile disassembly and inversion technique. The neoclitoris is formed from the dorsal glans penis; the vaginal lining is created with the penile and scroto-perineal flaps; and the labia majora are created with the scrotum. The urethra is shortened, spatulated, and everted to create the urethra, urethral meatus, and portions of the labia minora and vestibular lining.

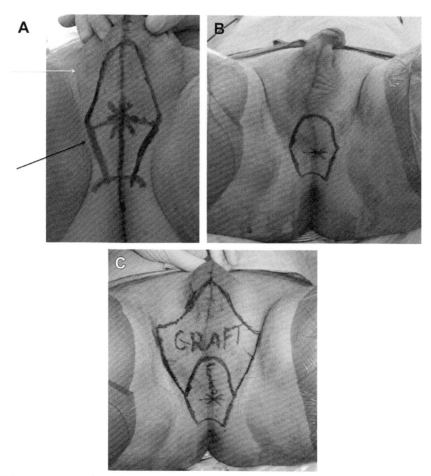

Fig. 5.8 (A) Preoperative markings for the scrotoperineal flap, when the flap is used to form the entire posterior vaginal wall. Note that (1) the flap borders, indicated by the black arrow, are maintained within the footprint of the lateral scrotum, indicated by the white arrow; (2) a "V"-shaped extension is designed at the planned level of the vaginal introitus; and (3) the base of the flap will maintain a broad subcutaneous pedicle without creating a rectangular appearance to the posterior labial commissure. The asterisk indicates the position of the central tendon, corresponding to the location of the vaginal introitus. (B) Preoperative markings for limited scrotoperineal flap. This flap is used when the distal penile skin remains tubularized. In this case, the scrotoperineal flap is shorter and only forms a portion of the posterior vaginal wall. The limited scrotoperineal flap is inset into the penile flap. (C) Limited scrotoperineal flap with full-thickness skin graft. In this case, the distal penile skin will remain tubularized, and additional scrotal skin will be harvested as a full-thickness skin graft.

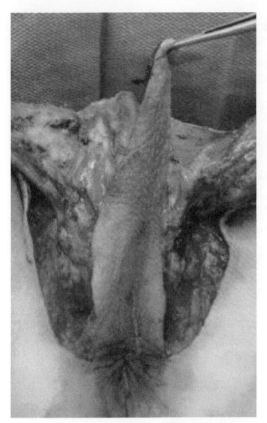

Fig. 5.9 Scrotoperineal flap is elevated. The flap should be thin, and its base should maintain a broad subcutaneous pedicle without creating a rectangular appearance to the posterior labial commissure.

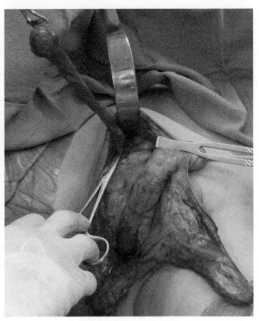

Fig. 5.11 Bilateral orchiectomies, including resection of the spermatic cords, are performed at the level of external inguinal ring. Resection of the spermatic cord at this level allows the ligated stump to retract into the inguinal canal and helps to prevent a palpable bulge.

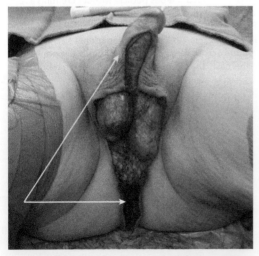

Fig. 5.10 The ventral penis is incised; the scrotoperineal flap is elevated and retracted posteriorly, and the testicles are exposed. The white arrow indicates the scroto-perineal flap, and the yellow arrow indicates the penile flap.

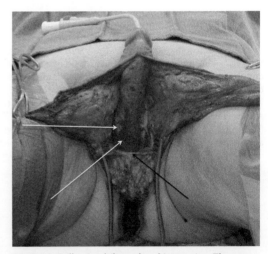

Fig. 5.12 Following bilateral orchiectomies. The superficial perineal musculature is exposed by retraction of the penile and scrotoperineal flaps. The bulbospongiosus muscle, indicated by the yellow arrow, overlies the corpora spongiosum; the ischiocavernosus muscles, indicated by the white arrow, overlie the corpora cavernosa, and the superficial transverse perinei muscle, indicated by the black arrow, inserts into the perineal body. The introitus is created at the location of the central tendon.

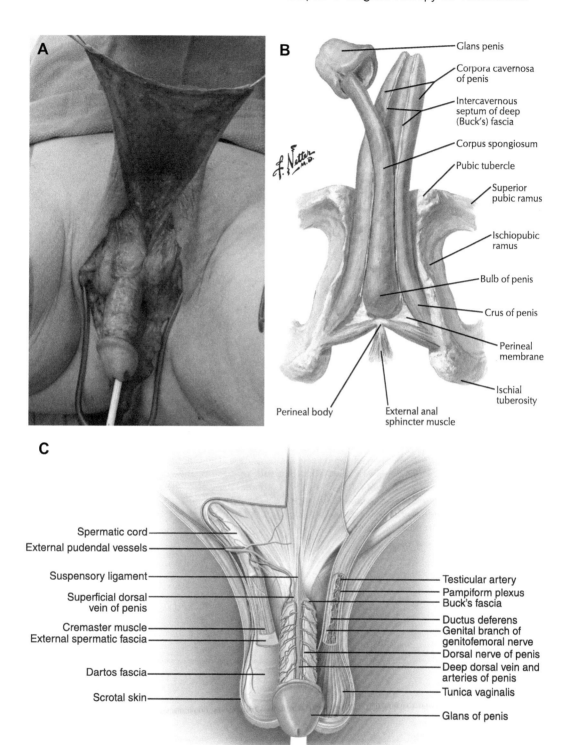

Fig. 5.13 (A) Penile degloving with elevation of the anteriorly based penile flap. This exposes the underlying corpora cavernosa dorsally, and the corpora spongiosum ventrally. (B and C) The glans penis represents an extension of the corpora spongiosum and is anatomically distinct from the corpora cavernosa. This allows the glans penis to be separated from the corpora cavernosa. The glans, elevated on the dorsal neurovascular pedicle, remains viable and innervated, and it will ultimately be used to create the neoclitoris. ([B] Copyright © 2016. Used with permission of Elsevier. All rights reserved. www.netterimages.com; and [C] From Schechter L. Surgery for gender identity disorder. In: Neligan PC, editor. Plastic surgery. 3rd edition. Philadelphia: Elsevier; 2013; with permission.)

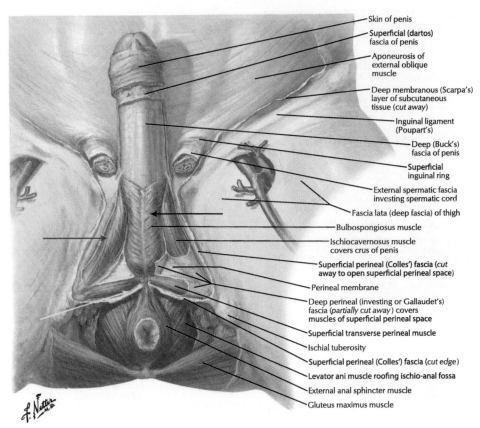

Fig. 5.14 Schematic of superficial perineal compartment musculature. The bulbospongiosus muscle, indicated by the black arrow, assists with emptying of the urethra and with erection of the corpora spongiosum and penis. The ischiocavernosus muscles, indicated by the red arrow, compress the crus of the penis, impedes venous return, and helps to maintain an erection. The superficial transverse perinei muscle, indicated by the yellow arrow, inserts into the perineal body. The superficial muscles are resected in order to widen the introitus. (Copyright © 2016. Used with permission of Elsevier. All rights reserved. www.netterimages.com.)

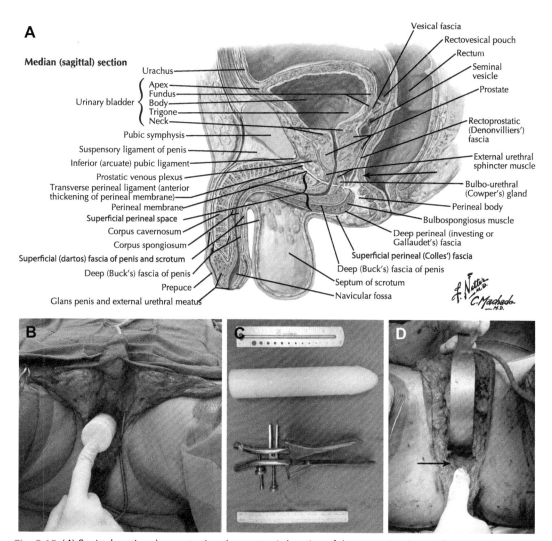

A

Median (sagittal) section

Vesical fascia
Rectovesical pouch
Rectum
Seminal vesicle
Prostate

Urachus

Urinary bladder
{ Apex
Fundus
Body
Trigone
Neck

Rectoprostatic (Denonvilliers') fascia

Pubic symphysis
Suspensory ligament of penis
Inferior (arcuate) pubic ligament
Prostatic venous plexus
Transverse perineal ligament (anterior thickening of perineal membrane)
Perineal membrane
Superficial perineal space
Corpus cavernosum
Corpus spongiosum
Superficial (dartos) fascia of penis and scrotum
Deep (Buck's) fascia of penis
Prepuce
Glans penis and external urethral meatus

External urethral sphincter muscle
Bulbo-urethral (Cowper's) gland
Perineal body
Bulbospongiosus muscle
Deep perineal (investing or Gallaudet's) fascia
Superficial perineal (Colles') fascia
Deep (Buck's) fascia of penis
Septum of scrotum
Navicular fossa

B   **C**   **D**

Fig. 5.15 (A) Sagittal section demonstrating the anatomic location of the neovagina (*arrow*) between the urethra, prostate, and bladder anteriorly and the rectum posteriorly. Dissection follows Denonvillier fascia. During dissection of the vaginal cavity, injury to the rectum may occur. (B and C) Development of the neovagina with dilator in place. (D) Retractor placed in the neovaginal cavity. Note the anal sphincter (*arrow*). The dissection of the vaginal cavity is performed in an extrasphincteric plane. ([A] Copyright © 2016. Used with permission of Elsevier. All rights reserved. www.netterimages.com.)

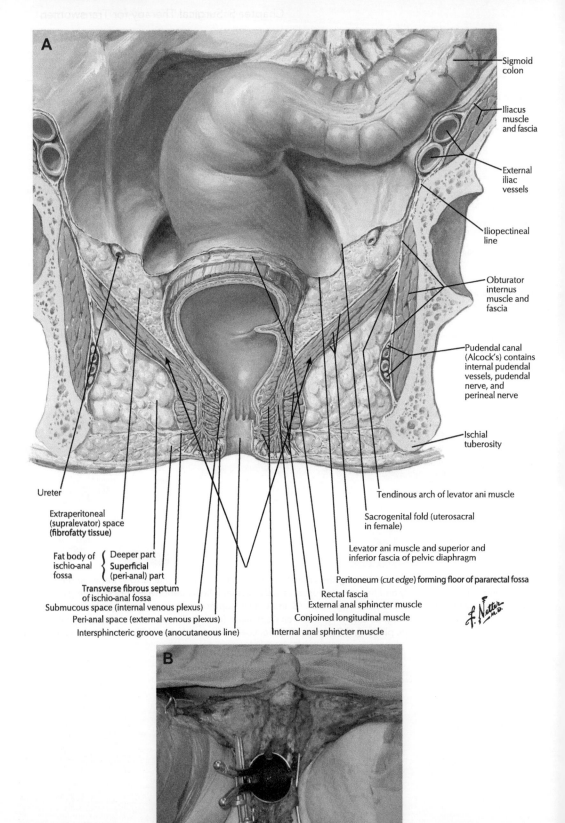

A

Sigmoid colon

Iliacus muscle and fascia

External iliac vessels

Iliopectineal line

Obturator internus muscle and fascia

Pudendal canal (Alcock's) contains internal pudendal vessels, pudendal nerve, and perineal nerve

Ischial tuberosity

Tendinous arch of levator ani muscle

Sacrogenital fold (uterosacral in female)

Levator ani muscle and superior and inferior fascia of pelvic diaphragm

Peritoneum (*cut edge*) forming floor of pararectal fossa

Rectal fascia
External anal sphincter muscle
Conjoined longitudinal muscle
Internal anal sphincter muscle

Ureter

Extraperitoneal (supralevator) space (fibrofatty tissue)

Fat body of ischio-anal fossa { Deeper part
Superficial (peri-anal) part

Transverse fibrous septum of ischio-anal fossa
Submucous space (internal venous plexus)
Peri-anal space (external venous plexus)
Intersphincteric groove (anocutaneous line)

B

Fig. 5.16 (*A*) Coronal section demonstrating levator ani. The release of the levator ani, indicated by the black arrows, aids with expansion of the neovaginal cavity. However, the natal male pelvis is narrower than that of the natal female pelvis. In some individuals, the bony pelvis may be a limiting factor in neovaginal width. (*B*) Vaginal speculum in place providing exposure for release of the levator ani muscles, bilaterally. The release of the levator ani allows expansion of the vaginal cavity. ([A] *Courtesy of* Netter medical illustration; with permission of Elsevier.)

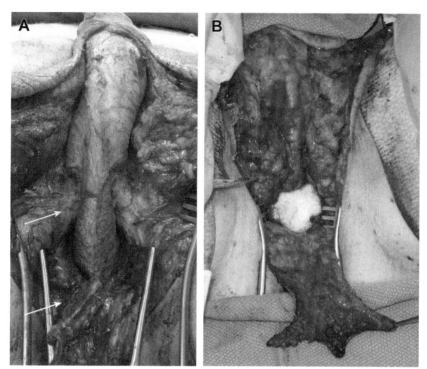

Fig. 5.17 (*A*) Elevation of the bulbospongiosus muscle, indicated by the white arrow, from the underlying corpora spongiosum. The corpora cavernosa are exposed following resection of the ischiocavernosus muscles, indicated by the yellow arrow. (*B*) Vaginal cavity developed (laparotomy sponge in place) and bulbospongiosus muscle resected.

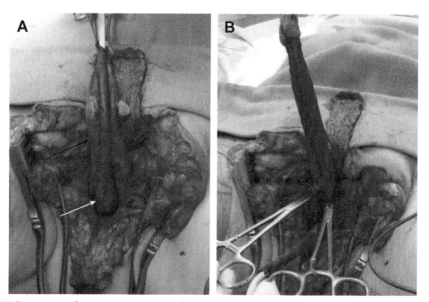

Fig. 5.18 (*A*) Separation of corpora spongiosum from corpora cavernosa. The white arrow indicates the corpora spongiosum, and the black arrow indicates the corpora cavernosa. (*B*) Clamps placed at base of corpora cavernosa in anticipation of resection. The glans, dissected on the dorsal neurovascular pedicle, is reflected anteriorly.

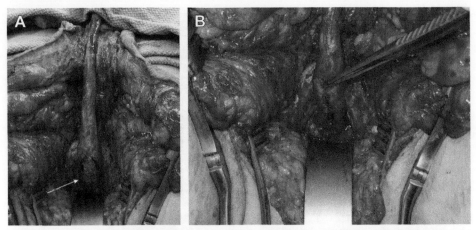

Fig. 5.19 (A) Marking, demonstrated by the arrow, indicates the planned area of resection of the corpora spongiosum. (B) Corpora spongiosum resected and oversewn. Resection of the corpora spongiosum allows expansion of the introitus. If excess erectile tissue remains, the tissue may become engorged upon arousal and obstruct entrance to the vaginal cavity.

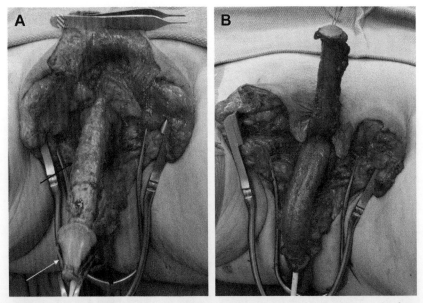

Fig. 5.20 (A) Design of the neoclitoris on the dorsal glans penis. The white arrow indicates the future neoclitoris designed from the glans penis. Dissection of the dorsal neurovascular pedicle incorporates buck fascia on the dorsal aspect of the corpora cavernosa. The black arrow indicates the position of the neurovascular pedicle. (B) Glans elevated on neurovascular pedicle.

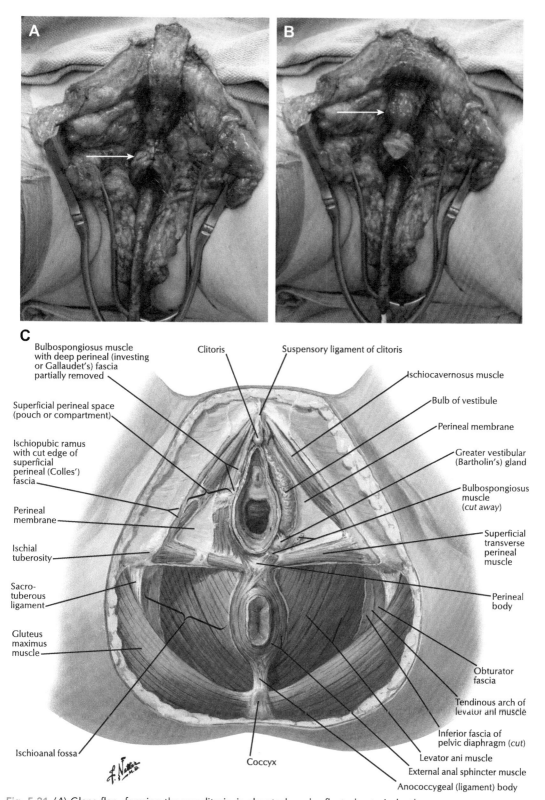

Fig. 5.21 (A) Glans flap, forming the neoclitoris, is elevated, and reflected anteriorly, the corpora cavernosa are resected and oversewn, and suture approximated (arrow). The urethra and corpora spongiosum are reflected caudally. (B) Positioning of the neoclitoris with suture fixation of (1) neoclitoral pedicle to anterior abdominal wall and (2) neoclitoris to underlying corpora cavernosa. The arrow indicates the pedicle of the glans flap. (C) The insert demonstrates the anatomy of the natal female clitoris. The natal female clitoris, like the natal male phallus, contains corpora cavernosa. The neoclitoris is constructed on top of the retained corporal bodies, simulating the natal female anatomy. ([C] Copyright © 2016. Used with permission of Elsevier. All rights reserved. www.netterimages.com.)

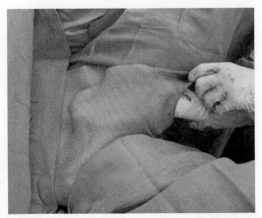

Fig. 5.22 Undermining and advancement of the abdominal skin in order to facilitate intravaginal positioning of the penile flap. The advanced abdominal skin flap is sutured to the anterior abdominal wall for stabilization.

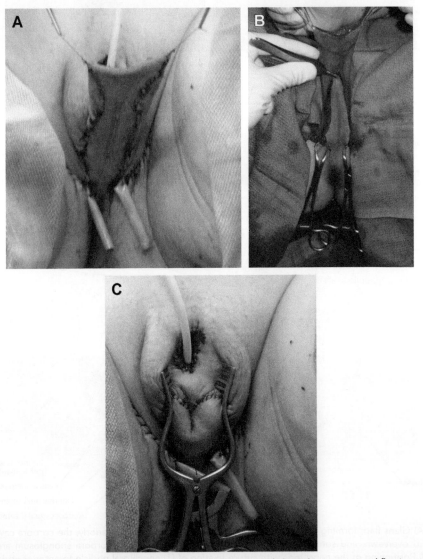

Fig. 5.23 (A) Creation of the skin-lined neovaginal cavity. The posteriorly based scrotoperineal flap is sutured to the anteriorly based penile flap. This creates the vascularized tube that will be used to form the neovaginal cavity. (B) Alternative inset with limited scroto-perineal flap. Limited scrotoperineal flap inset into tubularized penile flap. (C) Invagination of the penile and scrotoperineal flaps.

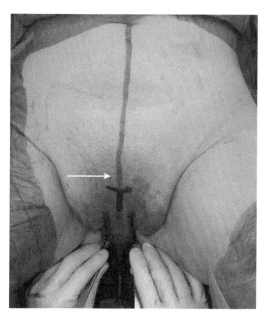

Fig. 5.24 "Y"-shaped incision for inset of the neoclitoris and urethra. The incision begins at the level of the pubic symphysis and extends inferiorly. The incision should be of sufficient length to allow exposure of the urethra, simulating the vestibular lining. The arrow indicates the position of the pubic symphysis.

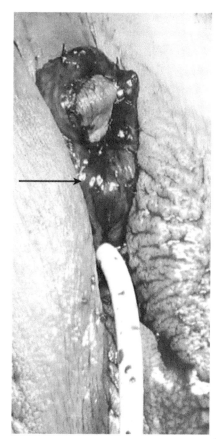

Fig. 5.26 Inset of the neoclitoris within the urethral flap. Sufficient exposure of the urethra creates a simulated vestibular lining, indicated by the arrow.

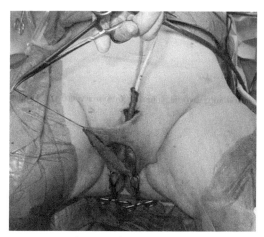

Fig. 5.25 Urethra transferred through the incision in the penile flap.

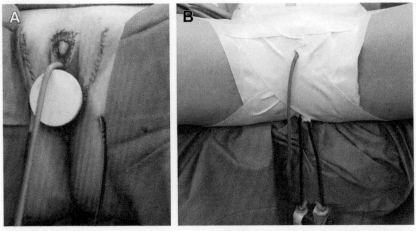

Fig. 5.27 (A) Placement of intravaginal stent, closed-suction drains, and urinary catheter. (B) Postoperative dressing in place. The intravaginal stent, drains, and urinary catheter will remain in place for approximately 4 to 5 days after surgery.

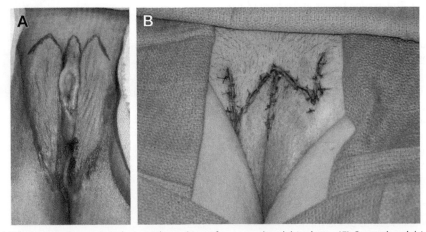

Fig. 5.28 (A) Postoperative vaginoplasty with markings for secondary labiaplasty. (B) Secondary labiaplasty performed following vaginoplasty. The labiaplasty provides convergence of the labia majora at the anterior commissure.

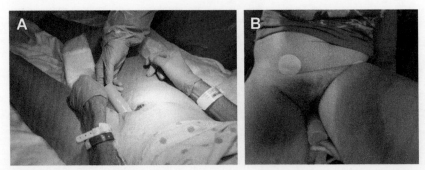

Fig. 5.29 (A) Patient instructed in postoperative vaginal dilation. (B) Patient performing postoperative vaginal dilation.

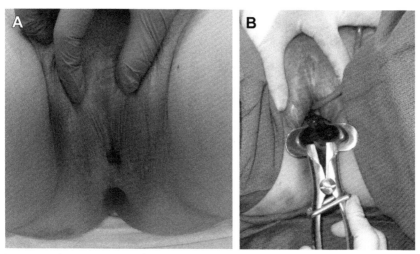

Fig. 5.30 (*A*) Patient with vaginal stenosis following vaginoplasty. (*B*) Preparation of perineum for intestinal vagino-plasty. The constricted introitus is released, allowing wide exposure of the vaginal cavity.

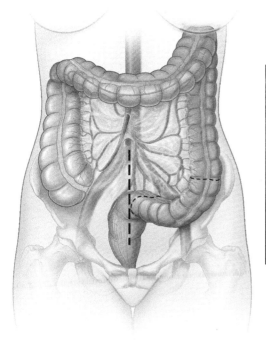

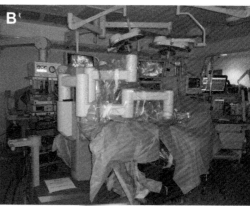

Fig. 5.31 (*A*) Anatomy and vascular supply of left colon. The intestinal segment will be transferred based on the mar-ginal artery as well as flow through the superior hemorrhoidal artery. (*B*) Robot docked. ([*A*] *From* Schechter L. Sur-gery for gender identity disorder. In: Neligan PC, editor. Plastic surgery. 3rd edition. Philadelphia: Elsevier; 2013; with permission.)

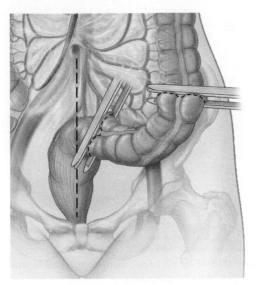

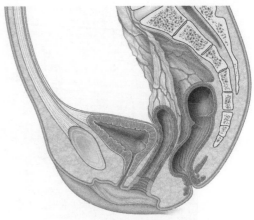

Fig. 5.34 Positioning of sigmoid colon. The sigmoid colon is inset between the urethra and bladder, anteriorly, and the rectum, posteriorly. (*From* Schechter L. Surgery for gender identity disorder. In: Neligan PC, editor. Plastic surgery. 3rd edition. Philadelphia: Elsevier; 2013; with permission.)

Fig. 5.32 Schematic demonstrating segment of sigmoid colon to be harvested for intestinal vaginoplasty. (*From* Schechter L. Surgery for gender identity disorder. In: Neligan PC, editor. Plastic surgery. 3rd edition. Philadelphia: Elsevier; 2013; with permission.)

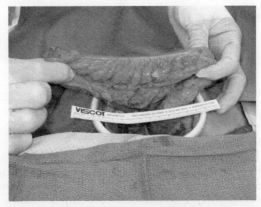

Fig. 5.33 Harvested segment of sigmoid colon in excess of 15 cm.

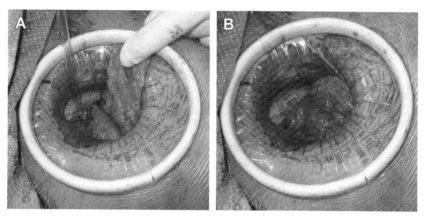

Fig. 5.35 (*A*) Colonic anastomosis for restoration of intestinal continuity. (*B*) Omentum interposed between the colonic anastomosis and the distal stump of the sigmoid vagina.

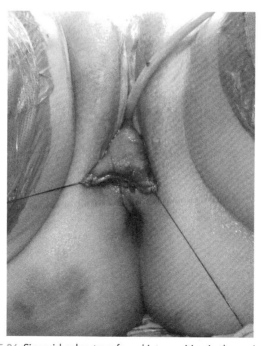

Fig. 5.36 Sigmoid colon transferred into position in the perineum.

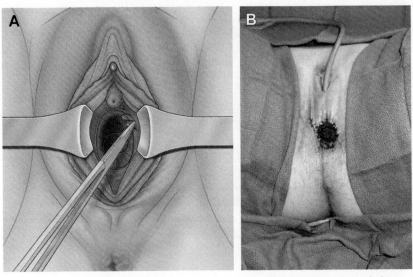

Fig. 5.37 (A) Postoperative sigmoid vaginoplasty. Sigmoid inset into perineal skin with single layer of absorbable sutures. (B) Postoperative sigmoid vaginoplasty (different patient). ([A] *From* Schechter L. Surgery for gender identity disorder. In: Neligan PC, editor. Plastic surgery. 3rd edition. Philadelphia: Elsevier; 2013; with permission.)

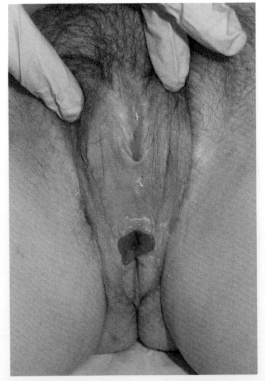

Fig. 5.38 Postoperative sigmoid vaginoplasty (different patient).

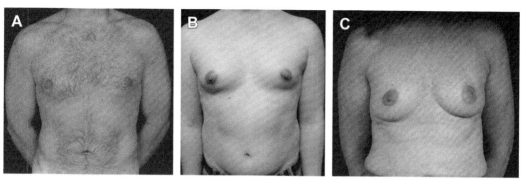

Fig. 5.39 Comparison of natal male, transfemale, and natal female breasts and chest wall. Note the differences in (1) the size and position of both the nipple and the areola, (2) the length between the nipple and the inframammary crease, (3) the prominence of the pectoralis major muscle, and (4) the chest wall width.

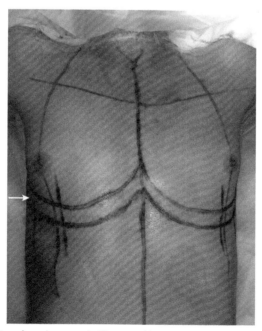

Fig. 5.40 Preoperative markings for subpectoral, silicone gel breast augmentation performed via an inframammary crease incision. The inframammary fold is lowered approximately 1 cm, indicated by the arrow. This allows the maximum point of implant projection to be positioned at the nipple level.

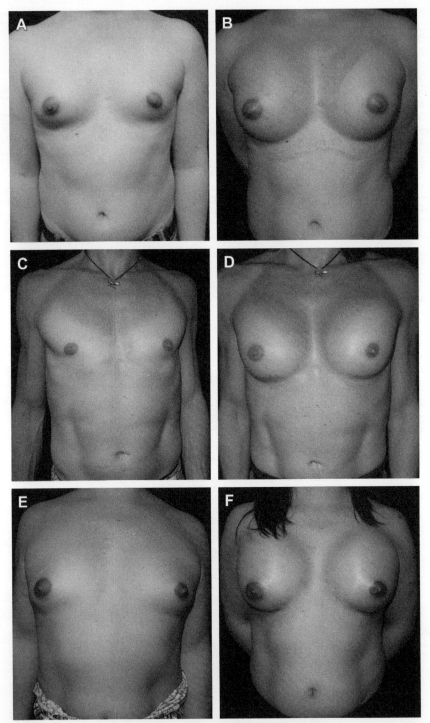

Fig. 5.41 (A and B) Preoperative and postoperative subpectoral, silicone gel breast augmentation performed via an inframammary crease incision. (C and D) Preoperative and postoperative subpectoral breast augmentation with form-stable implants performed via an inframammary crease incision. (E and F) Preoperative and postoperative subpectoral breast augmentation with form-stable implants performed via an inframammary crease incision.

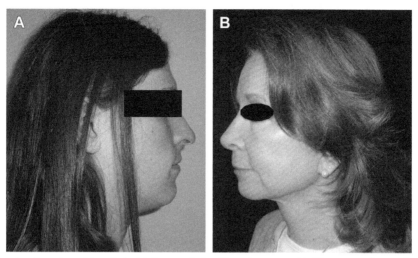

Fig. 5.42 Natal male and natal female facial characteristics. Note the supraorbital bossing in the natal male, and the more continuous forehead curvature in the natal female.

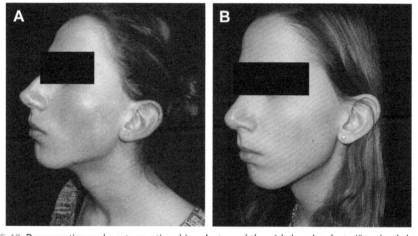

Fig. 5.43 Preoperative and postoperative rhinoplasty and thyroid chondroplasty ("tracheal shave").

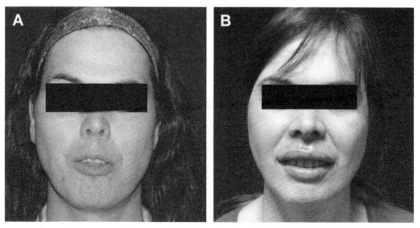

Fig. 5.44 Preoperative and postoperative upper lip shortening and lip augmentation. The lip is shortened through a "gull-wing"-shaped incision in the nostril sill.

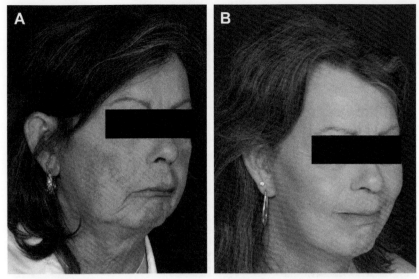

Fig. 5.45 Preoperative and postoperative upper eyelid blepharoplasty, facelift, and chemical peel.

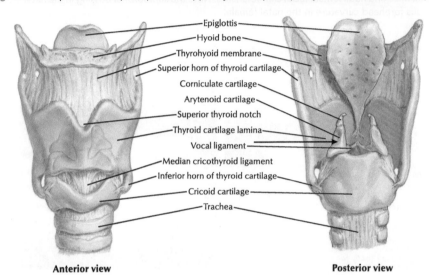

Epiglottis
Hyoid bone
Thyrohyoid membrane
Superior horn of thyroid cartilage
Corniculate cartilage
Arytenoid cartilage
Superior thyroid notch
Thyroid cartilage lamina
Vocal ligament
Median cricothyroid ligament
Inferior horn of thyroid cartilage
Cricoid cartilage
Trachea

Anterior view   **Posterior view**

Fig. 5.46 Anatomy of thyroid cartilage. Note the position of the thyroepiglottic ligament and the level of insertion of the vocal chords, indicated by the arrow. (Copyright © 2016. Used with permission of Elsevier. All rights reserved. www.netterimages.com.)

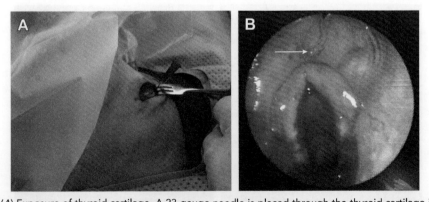

Fig. 5.47 (A) Exposure of thyroid cartilage. A 23-gauge needle is placed through the thyroid cartilage in order to assist with identification of the vocal cord insertion. (B) Fiberoptic visualization of the vocal cord insertion. A flexible fiberoptic scope is placed through an LMA by the anesthesiologist. A 23-gauge needle is placed through the thyroid cartilage, above the level of the vocal cord insertion. The arrow indicates the position of the needle. A position, approximately 2 to 3 mm above the insertion of the vocal cords, is marked on the external surface of the thyroid cartilage. This denotes the limit of cartilage resection and helps to maintain the stability of the vocal chords.

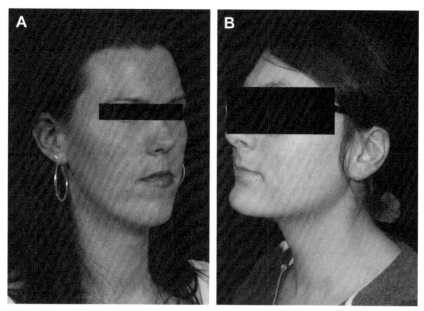

Fig. 5.48 Postoperative thyroid chondroplasty ("tracheal shave"), different patients.

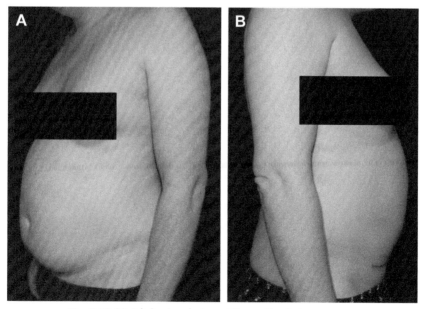

Fig. 5.49 Miniabdominoplasty and liposuction in transwoman.

REFERENCES

1. McIndoe AH, Bannister JB. An operation for the cure of congenital absence of the vagina. J Obstet Gynaecol Br Commonwealth 1938;5:490–4.

2. Edgerton M, Knorr N, Callison J. The surgical treatment of transsexual patients. Plast Reconstr Surg 1970;45(1):38–46.

3. Jones HW Jr, Schirmer HK, Hoopes JE. A sex conversion operation for males with transsexualism. Am J Obstet Gynecol 1968;100(1):101–9.

4. Pandya NJ, Stuteville OH. A one-stage technique for constructing female external genitalia in male transsexuals. Br J Plast Surg 1973;26(3):277–82.

5. Eldh J. Construction of a neovagina with preservation of the glans penis as a clitoris in male transsexuals. Plast Reconstr Surg 1993;91(5):895–900 [discussion: 901–3].

6. Hage JJ, Karim RB. Abdominoplastic secondary full-thickness skin graft vaginoplasty for male-to-female transsexuals. Plast Reconstr Surg 1998; 101(6):1512–5.

7. Karim RB, Hage JJ, Bouman FG, et al. The importance of near total resection of the corpus spongiosum and total resection of the corpora cavernosa in the surgery of male to female transsexuals. Ann Plast Surg 1991;26(6):554–6 [discussion: 557].

8. Rehman J, Melman A. Formation of neoclitoris from glans penis by reduction glansplasty with preservation of neurovascular bundle in male-to-female gender surgery: functional and cosmetic outcome. J Urol 1999;161(1):200–6.

9. Jarolim L. Surgical conversion of genitalia in transsexual patients. BJU Int 2000;85(7):851–6.

10. Krege S, Bex A, Lummen G, et al. Male-to-female transsexualism: a technique, results and long-term follow-up in 66 patients. BJU Int 2001;88(4):396–402.

11. Perovic SV, Stanojevic DS, Djordjevic ML. Vaginoplasty in male transsexuals using penile skin and a urethral flap. BJU Int 2000;86(7):843–50.

12. Malloy TR, Noone RB, Morgan AJ. Experience with the 1-stage surgical approach for constructing female genitalia in male transsexuals. J Urol 1976; 116(3):335–7.

13. Monstrey S, Hoebeke P, Dhont M, et al. Surgical therapy in transsexual patients: a multi-disciplinary approach. Acta Chir Belg 2001;101(5):200–9.

14. Kanhai RC, Hage JJ, Asscheman H, et al. Augmentation mammaplasty in male-to-female transsexuals. Plast Reconstr Surg 1999;104(2):542–9 [discussion: 550–1].

15. Laub D. Discussion: augmentation mammaplasty in male-to-female transsexuals. Plast Reconstr Surg 1999;104(2):550–1.

16. Ousterhout DK. Feminization of the forehead: contour changing to improve female aesthetics. Plast Reconstr Surg 1987;79(5):701–13.

17. Hage JJ, Vossen M, Becking AG. Rhinoplasty as part of gender-confirming surgery in male transsexuals: basic considerations and clinical experience. Ann Plast Surg 1997;39(3):266–71.

18. Hage JJ, Becking AG, de Graaf FH, et al. Gender-confirming facial surgery: considerations on the masculinity and femininity of faces. Plast Reconstr Surg 1997;99(7):1799–807.

19. Spiegel JH, Rodriguez G. Chondrolaryngoplasty under general anesthesia using a flexible fiberoptic laryngoscope and laryngeal mask airway. Arch Otolaryngol Head Neck Surg 2008;134(7):704–8.

20. Wolfort FG, Dejerine ES, Ramos DJ, et al. Chondrolaryngoplasty for appearance. Plast Reconstr Surg 1990;86(3):464–9 [discussion: 470].

21. Ettner R. The etiology of transsexualism. New York: The Haworth Press; 2007.

22. Lechien JR, Delvaux V, Huet K, et al. [Transgender voice and communication treatment: review of the literature]. Rev Laryngol Otol Rhinol (Bord) 2014; 135(2):97–103.

23. McNeill EJ. Management of the transgender voice. J Laryngol Otol 2006;120(7):521–3.

CHAPTER 6

Surgical Therapy for Transmen

CHEST SURGERY

Chest-wall contouring is an important, early surgical step for transmen and may help to facilitate their transition. The goals of chest surgery include the aesthetic contouring of the chest by removal of breast tissue and excess skin, reduction and repositioning of the nipple-areola complex when necessary, release of the inframammary crease, liposuction of the chest, and, when possible, minimization of chest scars and preservation of nipple sensitivity.[1]

Chest surgery in transmen presents an aesthetic challenge because of breast volume, breast ptosis, nipple-areola size and position, degree of skin excess, and potential loss of skin elasticity. Breast binding, commonly performed by transmen, may lead to the loss of skin elasticity, thereby necessitating significant amounts of skin removal (Fig. 6.1). Several surgical methods are used, and the choice of technique depends on the skin quality and elasticity, the degree of breast ptosis, and the position of the nipple-areola complex.[1] In addition, preservation of subcutaneous fat on the mastectomy skin flaps, preservation of the pectoralis and serratus fascia, release of the inframmary crease and sternal attachments, and contouring of the lateral chest wall are also important components of chest surgery and chest wall contouring. Preoperative breast imaging (ie, ultrasound or mammogram) is performed based on patient age, personal and family history, and physical examination.

Small, nonptotic breasts can often be treated with periareolar incisions ("limited incision"). In these cases, the nipple may be reduced by a wedge resection of the lower pole, but the areola is not repositioned. A small amount of tissue is left beneath the nipple-areola to preserve viability (Fig. 6.2). Circumareolar ("purse-string") or vertical incisions with free nipple-areola grafts can be used for larger breasts with mild ptosis requiring smaller amounts of skin removal (Fig. 6.3). Finally, traditional transverse inframammary crease incisions ("double incision") with free nipple-areola grafts may better serve individuals with larger breast volumes and increased breast ptosis requiring large amounts of skin removal (Fig. 6.4).

Nipple reduction is commonly used, often in conjunction with free nipple-areola grafts (Fig. 6.5). In addition, liposuction is frequently used for discontiguous undermining of the inframammary crease and lateral chest wall. Generally, free nipple-areola grafts, as opposed to the maintenance of the nipple-areola complex on a dermoglandular pedicle, are the preferred technique for nipple transposition so as to prevent residual breast fullness.

As with genital surgery, hormone therapy is discontinued 2 weeks before surgery. The patient is marked in the upright position. The relevant reference points include the inframammary crease, the midbreast meridian, the lateral border of the pectoralis major muscle, the axillary tail of the breast, midline, and the anticipated position of the nipple-areola complex (Fig. 6.6).

Before surgery, sequential compression devices are placed and intravenous antibiotics are administered. Following induction of general anesthesia, chemoprophylaxis for venous thromboembolism is administered subcutaneously (either fractionated or unfractionated heparin depending on institutional policies). With each of the operative techniques, the patient is positioned supine, with the arms abducted on foam rests with flexion at the elbow, and a lower-body forced-air warming blanket is placed. Draping should allow access to the surgical field from both above and below the upper extremity (Fig. 6.7). In addition, the patient is positioned and secured in anticipation of raising the back of the operating table in order to assess symmetry and guide placement of the nipple-areola grafts. The reference points are tattooed with methylene blue to aid with intraoperative identification (Fig. 6.8). If free nipple-areola grafts are to be performed, the nipple-areola complex is resized to a diameter of 2.5 to 3.0 cm. In addition, if a nipple reduction is required, a wedge resection of the lower pole of the nipple is performed (Fig. 6.9). The nipple-areola grafts are harvested, defatted, and placed in moist gauze sponges for later use (Fig. 6.10). When a skin resection is planned, regardless of the technique, the anticipated area of skin resection is incised in order to

61

facilitate breast removal (Fig. 6.11). The skin flaps are developed at the junction between the breast tissue and the subcutaneous fat (Fig. 6.12). The inframammary crease is undermined approximately 1 to 2 cm (Fig. 6.13). The medial dissection of the breast stops at the sternal border, and the perforating branches of the internal mammary artery are preserved, if possible. The lateral dissection proceeds subcutaneously over the serratus muscle, with preservation of the serratus fascia, and the breast is reflected off of the chest wall, with preservation of the pectoralis fascia (Fig. 6.14). Liposuction of the inframammary crease, the lateral chest, and the axillary tail is performed (Fig. 6.15). Fibrin sealant is placed in the cavity (Fig. 6.16); the patient is sat upright, and the skin flaps are tailored and inset (Fig. 6.17) in a layered fashion over a 15-French closed suction drain. Following resection, the breast tissue is marked and sent to pathology for routine examination.

In positioning the nipple-areolar complex, clinical judgment is used. In general, the nipple-areola is positioned medial to the lateral border of the pectoralis major muscle, approximately 1 to 2 cm above the inferior insertion of the pectoralis major muscle (Fig. 6.18). The nipple-areola is inset on a dermal bed, and a bolster dressing is placed (Fig. 6.19).

An elastic compression wrap remains in place for 4 to 5 days (Fig. 6.20A). At the time of the initial dressing change on postoperative day 4 or 5, the bolster is removed, and local care with a topical antimicrobial ointment is initiated. The compression wrap is continued for 3 weeks after surgery, followed by a compression shirt for an additional 3 weeks (Fig. 6.20B, C).

Secondary revisions related to the mastectomy scar and/or the nipple-areolar complex are not uncommon. Additional complications include, but are not limited to, hematoma, seroma, infection, delayed healing, loss of nipple grafts, asymmetry, and underresection and overresection of tissue leading to chest wall contour abnormalities.

GENITAL SURGERY FOR TRANSMEN
The goal of genital surgery in transmen may range from clitoral release (metoidioplasty), with or without urethral lengthening, to creation of a penis, capable of sexual penetration.[2] Similar to genital surgery for transwomen, transmen undergoing genital surgery discontinue their hormone therapy 2 weeks before surgery and complete a bowel preparation the day before surgery. Before surgery, sequential compression devices are placed and intravenous antibiotics are administered. Following

induction of general anesthesia, chemoprophylaxis for venous thromboembolism is administered subcutaneously (either fractionated or unfractionated heparin depending on institutional policies); the patient is positioned in the lithotomy position, and bony prominences are padded. For metoidioplasty procedures, the arms are abducted on foam rests with flexion at the elbows; an upper body forced-air surgical warming blanket is placed, and an indwelling urinary catheter is inserted under sterile conditions after the patient is prepared and draped. For phalloplasty procedures, a 325-mg aspirin suppository is administered, and the upper extremity chosen as the donor site is placed on a hand table, with a tourniquet applied to the upper arm.

Most transmen undergoing genital surgery will have undergone a hysterectomy and oophorectomy at least 3 months before either metoidioplasty or phalloplasty. For hysterectomy and oophorectomy procedures, either a laparoscopic or a vaginal approach is preferred. However, access for the vaginal route may be limited in nulliparous patients on testosterone therapy.

Metoidioplasty
Metoidioplasty, described in 1996 by Hage,[3] is an alternative to microsurgical or pedicled-flap phalloplasty in transmen. The term, coined by Laub, is based on the Greek prefix meta-, relating to change, and aidoio, relating to the genitals.[3] The procedure entails lengthening the hormonally hypertrophied (Fig. 6.21) clitoris by release of the suspensory ligament and resection of the ventral chordee. In order to allow for urination while standing, the natal female urethra is lengthened with the use of labia minora, vaginal musculomucosal flaps, and buccal mucosal grafts.[4] Although metoidioplasty may permit urination while standing, it does not allow placement of an erectile device, and it is unlikely that individuals undergoing metoidioplasty will be able to engage in penetrative intercourse. In addition, scrotal reconstruction following metoidioplasty positions the scrotum in a lateral, rather than an anterior, position. As such, patients may describe their testicles as being positioned "between their legs" rather than "in front of their legs." The metoidioplasty procedure is less complex compared with phalloplasty, avoids the disadvantage of additional scarring at remote donor sites, and may be converted to a phalloplasty at a later date, if desired. For some transmen, these considerations are sufficient to warrant the choice of metoidioplasty over phalloplasty.

The operative technique involves removal of the female genitalia with vaginectomy and colpocleisis (see vaginectomy/colpocleisis in the later phalloplasty section) concomitant with clitoral release, urethral lengthening, and scrotoplasty.[5] A distally based, anterior vaginal wall flap may be used in conjunction with a vestibular lining flap in order to reconstruct the proximal neourethra.[3] On the ventral aspect of the clitoris, the urethral plate is divided and dissected from the clitoral bodies. The division of the chordee allows for the release of the ventral clitoral curvature, permitting straightening and lengthening of the clitoris.[5] A suprapubic tube is placed for temporary urinary diversion.

The patient is positioned in the lithotomy position, and a lone star retractor is used for exposure of the urethra, clitoris, labia minora, and vagina (Fig. 6.22). An access incision, designed as a rectangular vestibular lining flap, is created between the native urethra and the virilized clitoris (Fig. 6.23). The vestibular lining flap is formed by 2 parallel incisions beginning at the native urethral meatus and extending along the vestibular lining toward the clitoris. Approximately one-third of the distance between the urethra and clitoris, a transverse incision communicates the 2 parallel incisions. The 2 parallel incisions are then extended to the clitoris and represent the medial incisions for the subsequent left and right labia minora flaps (Fig. 6.24).

The parallel incisions for the vestibular lining flap continue caudally, from the native urethral meatus, and extend intravaginally. These incisions, located along the anterior vaginal wall, are contiguous with the vaginal wall flap (Fig. 6.25). The vaginal flap is elevated as a musculomucosal flap, with its base at the urethral meatus (Fig. 6.26). These 2 flaps, the vestibular lining flap and the anterior vaginal wall flap, will be sutured to each other, forming the proximal urethra (Fig. 6.27).

The lateral and dorsal aspects of the corporal bodies are exposed through the aforementioned vestibular incisions and an incision located at the junction of the glans clitoris and the clitoral hood (Fig. 6.28). The plane of dissection follows the fascial layer covering the corporal bodies so as not to injure the vascular pedicle to the labia minora flaps. The skin is elevated to the pubic symphysis, and the suspensory ligament is identified. Division of the suspensory ligament remains at the discretion of the surgeon and depends on the length of the clitoris. The suspensory ligament may be left intact if there is adequate clitoral length, because division of this ligament may destabilize the clitoris. During this dissection, care is taken to preserve the clitoral neurovascular bundles located on the dorsum of the corporal bodies at approximately the 11 and 1 o'clock positions (Fig. 6.29).

Once the corporal bodies are anatomically defined, the ventral chordee is divided. Division of the chordee from the underlying corporal bodies allows straightening and advancement of the clitoris (Fig. 6.30).

The remainder of the urethral reconstruction is performed with bilateral labia minora flaps. The first flap is developed from the inner aspect of one side of the labia minora (left), and a second flap is developed from the contralateral labia minora (right) (Fig. 6.31). The 2 transposition flaps will overlap, creating a layered closure around the urethra. The left labia minora flap is outlined as a rectangle on the inner surface of the left labia minora, with the flap's medial border delineated by the previous vestibular incision. The outer, cutaneous, surface of the left labial flap is de-epithelialized. The contralateral right labial flap is elevated to allow subsequent mobilization over its left-sided counterpart. The cutaneous surface of the right-sided flap will be left intact, because this forms the ventral skin of the penile shaft (Fig. 6.32).

Construction of the urethra commences with anchoring of the distal margin of the vestibular lining flap to the corpora cavernosa (Fig. 6.33). A buccal mucosa graft is harvested, defatted, and sutured to the ventral corporal bodies with multiple quilting sutures (Figs. 6.34 and 6.35). The dimensions of the buccal graft correspond to the size of the defect created by the resection of the ventral chordee and typically measure approximately 1.5 cm × 6 cm (Fig. 6.36). Creation of the proximal urethra is completed by suturing the vaginal wall flap to the vestibular lining flap (Fig. 6.37).

The remainder of the urethra is fashioned using the previously elevated labia minora flaps. The left labial flap is shifted distally, transposed over the urinary catheter, sutured to the vestibular lining incisions on each side, and forms the ventral lining of the neourethra (Fig. 6.38). The contralateral right labial flap is transposed over the neourethra (left labia minora flap) and provides a layered closure as well as the ventral skin of the penile shaft (Figs. 6.39 and 6.40).

Scrotoplasty, constructed with bilateral labia majora flaps, is then performed. However, testicular implants are not placed at this time. A secondary surgical procedure is required for placement of the testicular implants so as to reduce the risk of infection and urethral complications (Fig. 6.41).

Additional masculinization of the lower abdominal and pubic areas may be performed with a mons resection. This procedure, performed through a Pfannenstiel incision, is designed to resect and reposition excess fatty tissue often found overlying the natal female pubis. Anchoring of Scarpa fascia to the rectus sheath aids with stabilization of the pubic tissue (Fig. 6.42). The mons resection is typically performed during placement of the testicular prostheses, so as not to communicate with the suprapubic tube, placed at the time of the initial metoidioplasty surgery. The mons resection helps to create the illusion of a longer phallus following metoidioplasty.

Patients are hospitalized for 2 to 3 days to allow for pain control, intravenous antibiotics, and incisional care (Box 6.1). Urination through the penis typically begins about 3 weeks after the procedure, following assessment of the urethral conduit. The suprapubic catheter is removed once the patient demonstrates effective transurethral voiding.

Complications following metoidioplasty include, but are not limited to, hematoma, delayed healing, infection, and urethral fistula and/or stricture.

Some individuals who have undergone metoidioplasty request subsequent conversion to a phalloplasty. In such circumstances, the glans penis, representing the former glans clitoris, is de-epithelialized and separated from the reconstructed urethra (Figs. 6.43 and 6.44). In addition, one of the dorsal clitoral nerves is harvested for later coaptation to the medial antebrachial cutaneous nerve of the forearm (Fig. 6.45). The glans-urethral construct is transposed subcutaneously and anchored in position to the pubic symphysis. The now redundant skin of the penile shaft, representing the former skin of the labia minora, is excised. If possible, the scrotum is

---

BOX 6.1
Postoperative orders: metoidioplasty

The patient is transferred directly to the hospital bed from the operating room (OR) table

Admit to Dr Schechter

Status postmetoidioplasty

Stable

Allergies:

Activity: Strict bed rest overnight, may be out of bed with assistance postoperative day 1

Nursing: Input/Output, spirometry 10 times/h, sequential compression devices at all times

Suprapubic tube to gravity drainage; do not remove urethral catheter; do not remove suprapubic catheter

Diet: Nothing by mouth overnight; advance to general diet postoperative diet number 1 after seen by Dr Schechter

Intravenous fluids: lactated Ringer at 100 mL/h. Change to Dextrose 5% 0.45 normal saline with 20 meq KCl at 80 mL/h postoperative day 1

Medication:

Piperacillin/tazobactam 3.375 g intravenously piggyback (IVPB) every 6 h (if allergic, ciprofloxacin 400 mg IVPB every 12 h and metronidazole 500 mg IV every 8 h, may need to add vancomycin 1 g IVPB every 12 [pharmacy to dose]) × 2 days

Patient-controlled analgesia (PCA) as ordered (morphine 1 mg with 12-min lockout, may substitute with dilaudid)

Metoclopramide 10 mg IVPB every 6 h

Enoxaparin 40 mg subcutaneously every day start postoperative day 1 after seen by Dr Schechter

Solifenacin succinate 5 mg orally twice a day

Bacitracin ointment at bedside

Laboratory tests: complete blood count (CBC), electrolytes on postoperative day 1

Dressing supplies:

Gauze pads at bedside

Petrolatum gauze at bedside

Abdominal pads at bedside

Suture removal kit at bedside

repositioned with anterior advancement of the previous scrotoplasty. The remainder of the procedure follows the principles of the phalloplasty outlined in the next section.

Phalloplasty

Phalloplasty represents the most complete genitoperineal transformation for transmen. Phalloplasty techniques may be divided into pedicled flaps and free flaps. Pedicle flaps transfer tissue, typically from the thigh, groin, or lower abdomen to reconstruct the penis, whereas free flaps involve the microsurgical transfer of tissue from a remote location.

The radial forearm free flap remains the gold standard for phallic reconstruction. This procedure transfers tissue, including the radial artery, venae comitantes, cephalic vein, and lateral and medial antebrachial cutaneous nerves, from the forearm to reconstruct the penis and urethra (Figs. 6.46 and 6.47). This flap allows the single-stage reconstruction of a sensate phallus and glans penis. Preoperative electrolysis of the volar, ulnar surface of the donor forearm may be required for depilation of what will become the penile urethra. Effective hair removal can take several months and should be completed at least 2 weeks before surgery. Potential drawbacks of this technique include the visibility of the donor site on the forearm, and the need for microsurgical skills.

The perineal reconstruction is performed with construction of the fixed, or membranous, urethra, from the vaginal and vestibular lining, as well as scrotal reconstruction with labia majora flaps (Fig. 6.48). Urethral complications, including both strictures and fistulae, are not uncommon, and additional, secondary procedures performed at a later date are required for placement of testicular implants and the erectile prosthesis.

Phalloplasty is performed with 2 surgical teams. One team performs the vaginectomy, colpocleisis, creation of the membranous urethra, scrotoplasty, and placement of a suprapubic tube, while the second team harvests and shapes the forearm flap, then closes the forearm donor site.

The vaginectomy is performed by removal of the vaginal epithelium from the fibromuscular vaginal wall (Fig. 6.49). With the patient in the lithotomy position, a lone star retractor is placed, and the subepithelial space is injected with xylocaine with epinephrine. The vaginal epithelium of the distal posterior midline is incised from the midvagina to the level of the perineal skin. This incision facilitates access to the proximal one-third of the vagina, and additional access may be provided by release of the paramedian epithelium

as well. A combination of sharp dissection with scissors and electrocautery is used to remove the epithelium laterally, up to the vaginal apex. Anterior dissection of the midproximal vagina is performed. Dissection in the anterior-lateral sulci at the midvaginal level may be associated with an increased risk of bleeding due to the proximity of the vaginal venous plexus. The distal epithelium, including the hymenal tissue, is removed up to the margin of the paraurethral sulci bilaterally, and the urethral meatus anteriorly. If a vaginal flap will be used in creation of the proximal urethra, the corresponding portion of the vagina is left intact (Fig. 6.50). Interrupted mattress sutures of 2-0 Vicryl are then used to close the vaginal space and perform the colpocleisis.

The fixed, or membranous, portion of the urethra is created by tubularization of the vestibular lining, located between the native urethral orifice and the virilized clitoris. Two parallel incisions are made from the native urethral orifice and extend to the clitoris. The distal, dorsal aspect of the vestibular lining is spatulated in order to enlarge the anastomosis between the membranous and penile urethrae. When a vaginal flap is needed for construction of the proximal portion of urethra, the vestibular incisions extend intravaginally and communicate with the planned vaginal flap (Figs. 6.51 and 6.52). The vaginal flap is elevated and left in situ, in anticipation of approximation to the vestibular lining (Fig. 6.53).

The vestibular incisions allow access to and exposure of the lateral aspect of the corporal bodies. The dorsal surface of the corporal bodies is exposed through an incision at the junction of the glans clitoris and clitoral hood (Figs. 6.54 and 6.55). The labial skin is dissected to the pubic symphysis, and care is taken to preserve the dorsal clitoral neurovascular bundles. Following exposure of the corporal bodies, the glans clitoris is injected with 1% xylocaine with epinephrine and de-epithelialized. One of the dorsal clitoral neurovascular bundles is harvested and tagged for subsequent neurorrhaphy. The nerve bundle on the side opposite of the planned vascular anastomosis is chosen. Reconstruction of the membranous urethra is completed with tubularization of the vestibular lining over an 18-French urinary catheter (Figs. 6.56–6.60).

The donor site incision, taking the shape of a flattened "omega (Ω)," is designed overlying the pubic symphysis (Fig. 6.61). A subcutaneous tunnel is then created between the donor site incision and the degloved clitoris (Fig. 6.62). The clitoris is transposed subcutaneously and fixed to the pubic bone (Fig. 6.63). Fixation of the clitoris aids with stabilization of the urethral construct.

The perineal portion of the surgery proceeds with resection of the labia minora and scrotoplasty so as to eliminate the remaining vestiges of the female anatomy. The labia minora are resected in their entirety, and the scrotoplasty is performed with medial transposition of the labia majora. Incisions on the lateral border of the labia majora facilitate their mobilization to a position anterior to the legs (Fig. 6.64). Pelvic floor reconstruction is completed by suture approximation of the superficial pelvic musculature and layered skin closure.

Interrupted sutures are preplaced in the os of the reconstructed membranous urethra, now located at the level of the pubic symphysis (Fig. 6.65). These sutures will be used in completing the distal anastomosis between the penile urethra of the forearm flap and the membranous urethra created from the tubularized vestibular lining. At this point, the patient is taken out of the lithotomy position, placed in the supine position, and reprepared.

Dissection of the recipient vessels begins with an incision, extended obliquely from the donor site incision, along the groin crease (Fig. 6.66). The superficial femoral artery, great saphenous vein, superficial inferior epigastric vein, superficial circumflex iliac vein, and ilioinguinal nerve are exposed. Vessel loops are used to encircle the superficial femoral artery, and the great saphenous is clamped proximally and divided distally. The ilioinguinal nerve is identified exiting the superficial inguinal ring and traveling with the round ligament. The nerve is transected distally and tagged for later neurorrhaphy (Fig. 6.67).

Flap harvest on the forearm begins with performance of an Allen's test. A cutdown is performed at the wrist; the radial artery is identified and occluded with a microvascular clamp, and a Doppler signal to the thumb is confirmed. The extremity is elevated, but not exsanguinated, allowing subsequent identification of the superficial venous system. The tourniquet is inflated, and dissection begins in the proximal forearm. The cephalic and median antebrachial veins are identified, and the lateral and medial antebrachial cutaneous nerves are dissected. The lateral antebrachial cutaneous nerve typically runs adjacent to the cephalic vein, and the anterior branch of the medial antebrachial cutaneous nerve typically runs adjacent to the median antebrachial vein (Fig. 6.68). The nerves are transected proximally and tagged for later coaptation to the ilioinguinal and dorsal clitoral nerves, respectively. A "tube-within-a-tube" technique is used to create the neophallus. The urethra is created from tubularization of the ulnar border of the flap, and the skin of the penile shaft is created from the skin of the radial border of the flap. An intervening strip of skin between the ulnar and radial portions of the flap is de-epithelialized in order to provide a layered closure overlying the penile urethra (Fig. 6.69). Multiple superficial veins are harvested, including the cephalic vein, incorporating the perforating branch of the deep venous system from the venae comitantes, and the median antebrachial vein (Fig. 6.70). The basilic vein is typically left in situ to aid with venous drainage of the nonharvested forearm skin.

Most often, flap elevation occurs in the suprafascial plane over the muscle bellies, and the paratenon overlying the distal tendons is preserved. During dissection of the radial border of the flap, the sensory branch of the radial nerve is identified and preserved. The radial artery is dissected to its takeoff from the brachial artery so as to allow maximum pedicle length for the arterial anastomosis. The venous dissection incorporates the perforating branch between the venae comitantes and cephalic vein (Fig. 6.71).

Following flap harvest, the penile urethra is tubularized over an 18- to 20-French urinary catheter, and the skin of the shaft is closed in a layered fashion. A glansplasty is performed by elevation of a distally based flap located approximately 3 cm from the distal border of the forearm flap. The glans is further defined by construction of the coronal ridge, and placement of a skin graft at the donor site of the distal flap harvest (Fig. 6.72).

The phallus is transferred to its position on the pubic symphysis (Fig. 6.73), and the urethral anastomosis is performed first. The preplaced urethral sutures, located in the distal os of the membranous urethra, are sutured to the penile urethra, incorporating the full thickness of the penile urethral skin.

Before occlusion of the femoral artery, a heparin bolus is administered. In addition, the patient is maintained on a heparin drip during the performance of the anastomoses, and a heparin solution consisting of 500 U/mL is used for intraluminal irrigation. The arterial anastomosis is performed first, in an end-to-side fashion, between the radial artery and the superficial femoral artery. Typically 2 or 3 venous anastomoses are performed in an end-to-end fashion between the cephalic and greater saphenous veins and the antebrachial vein(s) and superficial inferior epigastric and superficial circumflex iliac veins. When possible, a venous coupler is used. The neurorrhaphies are then completed between the lateral antebrachial cutaneous and ilioinguinal nerve and the medial antebrachial and dorsal clitoral nerves (Fig. 6.74A). Nerve wraps are placed over the neurorrhaphy (Fig. 6.74B). Placement of Penrose drains in each groin and layered closure of the skin complete the procedure (Fig. 6.75).

Closure of the forearm donor site is performed by reapproximation of the muscle bellies over a closed suction drain. A skin graft may be applied to the forearm donor site, or, alternatively, a bilayer wound matrix may be placed (Fig. 6.76A). If a wound matrix is used, a skin graft is performed at a later date. Most often, negative-pressure wound therapy (NPWT) in conjunction with a topical antimicrobial dressing is used to dress the forearm donor site (Fig. 6.76B). A light compression wrap is then applied (Fig. 6.76C).

Postoperatively, patients are maintained on a variable duration of bed rest with both transurethral and suprapubic catheters. The phallus is maintained in a vertical position with a soft gauze dressing (Fig. 6.77). Both mechanical and chemoprophylaxis are used for venous thromboembolism prophylaxis; aspirin 81 mg is administered daily, and flap monitoring is performed with a handheld Doppler. Range of motion is initiated on the donor forearm on postoperative day 1, and the negative pressure dressing is changed on postoperative day 4 or 5. Following the initial dressing change, the negative pressure dressing is changed at 2- to 3-day intervals using a topical antimicrobial dressing. The patient is typically discharged from the hospital on postoperative day 9 or 10 (Box 6.2).

If a wound matrix was used on the forearm donor site, the patient returns to the operating room after approximately 2 weeks for placement of a skin graft (Fig. 6.78). NPWT may be used to dress the skin graft, and the initial dressing change is performed on postoperative day 3 or 4. Routine forearm dressing changes are instituted with a topical antimicrobial ointment and a compression wrap. After approximately 4 to 6 weeks, compression garments may be placed on the forearm to assist with scar maturation (Fig. 6.79).

Urination through the penile urethra may begin as early as 3 weeks following phalloplasty. Manual milking of the urethra may be required to assist with complete drainage of residual urine (Fig. 6.80).

Perhaps the next most used technique for phalloplasty is the use of tissue from the thigh, known as the anterolateral thigh (ALT) flap. Similar to the forearm technique, tissue, including the lateral femoral cutaneous nerve, may be transferred from the thigh to construct the penis. Depending on the individual's distribution of subcutaneous fat, a tube-within-a-tube technique may be used, or a second flap may be required for urethral reconstruction. The ALT flap may require secondary debulking procedures because of the amount of subcutaneous fat. As with the forearm flap, the urethra is formed by a skin-lined tube. As such, preoperative depilation may be required for the portions of the flap used for urethral construction.

A musculocutaneous latissimus dorsi (MLD) flap may also be used for phalloplasty. Two downsides of this flap are the lack of a sensory nerve in the donor tissue and potential bulk of the constructed phallus. Other phalloplasty techniques involve pedicled abdominal or groin flaps (Table 6.1).

Testicular implants and penile prostheses can be placed at a secondary procedure. Although the testicular implants may be placed as early as 3 months following phalloplasty, the penile prosthesis is typically placed 9 to 12 months after the phalloplasty. This amount of time allows the development of protective sensation, which is important for retention of the erectile device.

Before placement of the testicular implants, and depending on the volume of the scrotal sac, remote fill tissue expanders may be placed as an interval procedure (Fig. 6.81). Remote fill tissue expanders may aid with expansion of the scrotal sac, if necessary, and allows placement of larger testicular implants. The implants are typically suture stabilized to the base of the scrotum so as to minimize the risk of displacement (Figs. 6.82 and 6.83).

The final stage of penile reconstruction involves placement of the erectile device. Although both malleable and inflatable prostheses are available, neither device is specifically designed for placement in a flap phalloplasty. As such, anchoring of the prosthesis can be a challenge and often requires fixation to the pubic bone. Anchoring of the prosthesis may be performed with suture fixation to the periosteum of the pubis, or, alternatively, bone anchoring. In addition, the prostheses can be wrapped with an acellular dermal matrix to help form a "pseudo corpora cavernosa."

Although the malleable device is less mechanically complicated, its permanent rigidity can result in erosion of the prosthesis through the skin or urethra (Fig. 6.84A). The device is soaked in antibiotic solution and cut to appropriate length, and the tip is placed (Fig. 6.84B–E).

When choosing the inflatable device, either a 2-piece or 3-piece implant is available. With the 3-piece device, the pump is placed in the scrotal sac and serves the purpose of a testicular implant. The reservoir is placed in a retroperitoneal position. Depending on the dimensions of the phallus,

BOX 6.2
Postoperative orders: phalloplasty

The patient is transferred directly to the hospital bed from the OR table

Admit to Dr Schechter

Status post-phalloplasty

Stable

Allergies:

Activity: Strict bed rest; penis to remain upright, do not manipulate (R/L) leg, (R/L) leg to remain flexed at hip and knee, do not abduct (R/L) lower extremity

Patient may ambulate on postoperative day (____) after seen by Dr Schechter

Nursing: Input/Output, spirometry 10×/h, sequential compression devices at all times, drain (R/L) upper extremity

Suprapubic tube to gravity drainage, no suppositories

Do not remove urethral catheter, do not remove suprapubic catheter

Bair hugger over perineum

Diet: Nothing by mouth (may start clear liquids postoperative day 1 after seen by Dr Schechter and general diet postoperative day 2 after seen by Dr Schechter)

Flap check: every 30 min × 6 h, then hourly

Intravenous fluids: lactated Ringer at 100 mL/h. Change to dextrose 5% 0.45 normal saline with 20 meq KCl at 80 mL/h postoperative day 1

Medication:

Piperacillin/tazobactam 3.375 g IVPB every 6 h (if allergic ciprofloxacin 400 mg IVPB every 12 h and metronidazole 500 mg IV every 8 h, may need to add vancomycin 1 g IVPB every 12 h [pharmacy to dose]) × 3 days

PCA as ordered (morphine 1 mg with 12-min lockout or dilaudid)

Metoclopramide 10 mg IVPB every 6 h

Enoxaparin 40 mg subcutaneously every day start postoperative day 1 after seen by Dr Schechter

Aspirin 81 mg daily, beginning postoperative day 1

Solifenacin succinate 5 mg orally twice a day may be added when taking orally

Bacitracin ointment at bedside

Laboratory tests: CBC, electrolytes, prothrombin time/partial thromboplastin time on arrival in intensive care unit and postoperative day 1

CBC, electrolytes postoperative day 2

NPWT to (R/L) upper extremity; physical therapy to change dressing postoperative day 4 and begin every 2- to 3-d dressing with Acticoat and NPWT. Patient to be discharged with NPWT.

Occupational therapy to begin range of motion on (R/L) upper extremity postoperative day 2

Biopatch on suprapubic tube changed postoperative days 4 and 7

Dressing supplies:

Gauze pads at bedside

Petrolatum gauze at bedside

Abdominal pads at bedside

2″ silk tape at bedside

Suture removal kit at bedside

Postoperative days 4 and 7 vac change to forearm with Acticoat

TABLE 6.1
Comparison of phalloplasty techniques

	RFAFF (Radial Forearm Free Flap)	ALT	MLD
Donor site	–	+/–	+
Urethra	+	+/–	+/–
Glans	+	–	–
Sensation	+	+	–
Prosthesis	–	+/–	+
Stages	2	2 (plus debulking)	3
	Donor site visibility Vascularized urethra in single stage Preoperative depilation Refined glans Lateral and medial antebrachial cutaneous nerve	Donor site concealed but requires graft May require second flap for urethra due to bulk Preoperative depilation Secondary glans shaping Lateral femoral cutaneous nerve May require secondary debulking procedures	Direct closure of donor site possible Second flap for urethra with staged urethral reconstruction Less refinement Insensate May require secondary debulking procedures

either a single or a double rod may be chosen (Figs. 6.85 and 6.86).

After-Discharge Care

Following metoidioplasty or phalloplasty, testosterone is resumed when ambulation is initiated. Patients should wear loose fitting clothing and avoid lifting more than 10 to 15 pounds for 6 weeks following surgery. Patients who undergo phalloplasty should place their penis upward, against the lower abdomen, while ambulating. In addition, topical antimicrobial ointment with nonadherent gauze and a light compression wrap is applied to the donor forearm for approximately 3 weeks. After 3 weeks, patients discontinue the antimicrobial ointment and apply moisturizing lotion to the skin graft twice daily. A compression garment can be worn beginning approximately 3 weeks after the skin graft, and it can be continued for approximately 3 to 6 months.

Patients are discharged with a suprapubic catheter. Before removing the catheter, the lower urinary tract is evaluated. A retrograde urethrogram may be performed to visualize the posterior urethra. Alternatively, in order to obtain both dynamic and functional images, contrast dye can be injected into the bladder via the suprapubic tube, and radiographs can be taken during micturition (Fig. 6.87). If abnormality is noted, cystoscopy can be used for further assessment.

Following metoidioplasty and phalloplasty, patients who travel are encouraged to remain in the area following discharge from the hospital. Those undergoing metoidioplasty and phalloplasty should stay approximately 5 to 7 days.

Complications

Complications following phalloplasty can be divided into early and late categories. Early complications tend be flap-related and include delayed wound healing and flap failure (Fig. 6.88). Additional early complications include venous thromboembolism, bleeding, and infection. Most late complications are urologic in nature and are discussed in detail later. Other late complications can be related to the erectile prosthesis; these include erosion, either through the shaft skin or urethra, dislodgement, and mechanical failure. Furthermore, disruption of the neurorrhaphy can occur during placement of the prosthesis, resulting in loss of sensation to the phallus.

Urethral complications

Urethral problems occur commonly after phalloplasty,[6] and additional procedures may be required. Complications include urinary tract infection, urethrocutaneous fistula, urethral stricture, urethral diverticula, and hair within the reconstructed urethra. Symptoms may include a weak urinary stream, leakage of urine from the penile shaft or scrotum, dysuria, urinary frequency, incomplete emptying, and inability to urinate.

Urinary tract infections. Urinary tract infections and colonization of indwelling catheters are common and can be difficult to manage. Symptoms include bladder spasms, suprapubic pain, dysuria, fever, hematuria, and malaise. Antibiotic therapy should be guided based on culture results.

Meatal stenosis. Meatal stenosis can range from mild, incomplete forms to complete obliteration (Fig. 6.89). For mild stenosis, dilation techniques, such as male urethral Van Buren sounds, balloon dilation,[7] or, in compliant patients, self-calibration of the urethral meatus with a catheter, can be used.[8]

Urethral strictures. Urethral strictures can occur at the anastomotic sites or along the length of the reconstructed urethra and can be partial or complete. Management includes both endoscopic and open techniques.

Endoscopic management, using urethral dilation or direct visual internal urethrotomy with laser or cold knife,[9] may be appropriate for incomplete, short segment strictures located at the anastomotic sites (Fig. 6.90).[10] For complete urethral obliteration and/or long segment or recurrent strictures, single-, or 2-stage urethroplasty with buccal mucosa grafts may be required (Fig. 6.91). Two to 3 weeks after urethroplasty, retrograde and anterograde urethrography is performed. If the individual voids well through the urethra, if there is minimal or no postvoid residual, and if there is no defect on urethrogram, remaining catheters are removed.

Urethrocutaneous fistula. Fistulous tracts may require evaluation with a urethrogram and/or a urethroscopy (Fig. 6.92). If there is sufficient local tissue and no infection, the fistula tract can be excised and reapproximated around a catheter in a single stage. A urethrogram is performed 2 to 3 weeks later, and, if no abnormality is seen, and if the patient is able to void with minimal or no residual, the catheter is removed.

Alternatively, for fistulae requiring staged procedures, a buccal mucosa graft is placed at the time of fistula excision (Figs. 6.93 and 6.94). Approximately 6 months later, the urethra is closed in a layered fashion over a catheter. A urethrogram is performed 2 to 3 weeks later, and, if no abnormality is seen, and if the patient is able to void with minimal or no residual, the catheter is removed.

Urethral hair or residual suture. Urethral reconstruction using hair-bearing tissue can cause stone formation,[11] reinforcing the importance of adequate preoperative depilation. In addition, use of long-lasting suture, such as polydioxanone, can lead to suture granulomas (Fig. 6.95). These issues may be treated with endoscopic techniques.

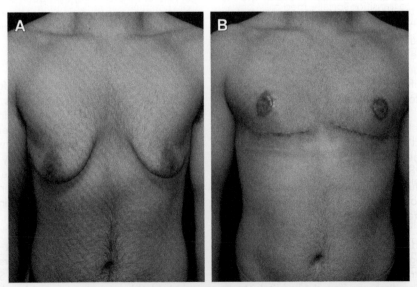

Fig. 6.1 (A) Preoperative photograph of a patient undergoing double-incision chest surgery. Preoperatively, note the degree of breast ptosis and the loss of skin elasticity. In addition, the nipple-areola complex requires reduction and repositioning. (B) Postoperative double-incision chest surgery with free nipple-areola grafts.

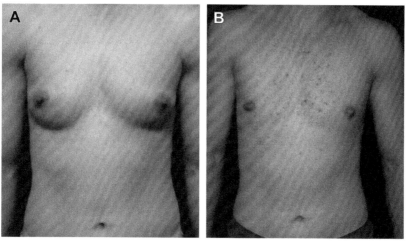

Fig. 6.2 Preoperative and postoperative photographs of patient undergoing limited incision chest surgery, including nipple reduction.

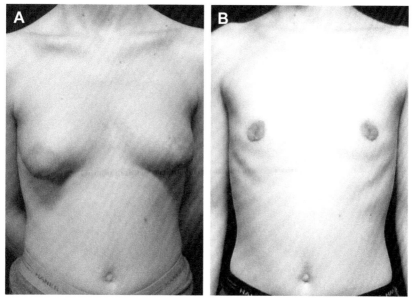

Fig. 6.3 Preoperative and postoperative photographs of patient undergoing purse-string chest surgery with free nipple-areola grafts and nipple reduction.

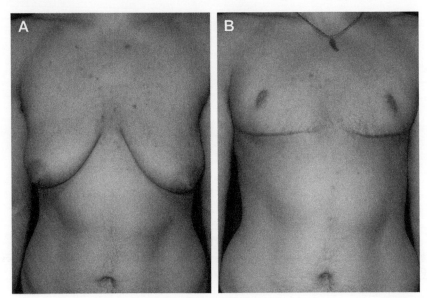

Fig. 6.4 (A) Preoperative photograph of patient undergoing double-incision chest surgery with free nipple-areola grafts and nipple reduction. (B) Postoperative photograph following double-incision chest surgery with free nipple-areola grafts and nipple reduction.

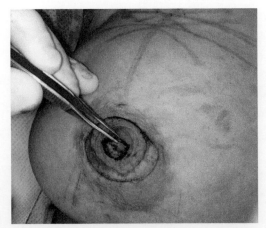

Fig. 6.5 Nipple reduction performed in conjunction with free nipple-areola graft. The nipple is resized to 30 mm, and a wedge resection of the lower pole of the nipple is performed.

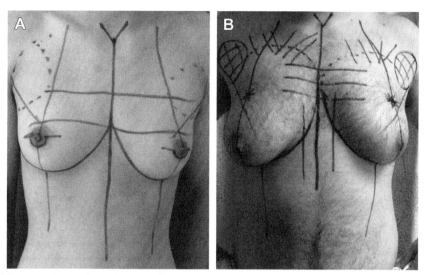

Fig. 6.6 (A) Preoperative markings for limited incision chest surgery, including midbreast meridian, inframammary crease, midline, axillary tail, and lateral border of pectoralis major. For limited incision approaches, the areola is not repositioned. (B) Preoperative markings for double-incision chest surgery with free nipple-areola grafts, including midbreast meridian, inframammary crease, axillary tail, lateral border of pectoralis major, midline, and the anticipated position of the nipple-areola complex. The nipple-areola complex is positioned medial to the lateral border of the pectoralis major muscle, approximately 1 to 2 cm above the inferior insertion of the pectoralis major muscle.

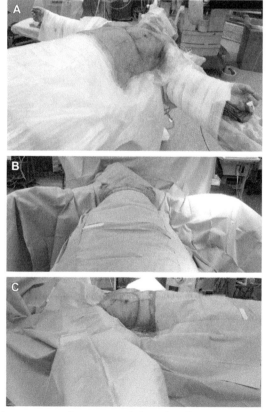

Fig. 6.7 (A) Positioning for chest surgery. The arms are abducted on foam rests, flexed at the elbow, and wrapped. A lower-body forced-air warming blanket is placed. (B and C) Draping allows access both above and below the upper extremities.

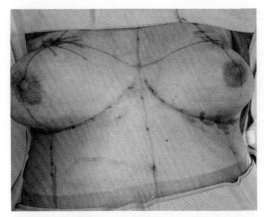

Fig. 6.8 Intraoperative markings tattooed with methylene blue, including midbreast meridian, inframammary crease, lateral border of pectoralis major muscle, midline, and the anticipated position of the nipple-areola complex.

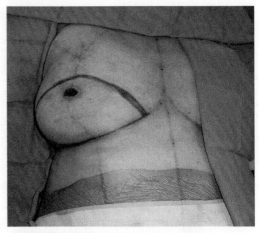

Fig. 6.11 Planned area of skin resection.

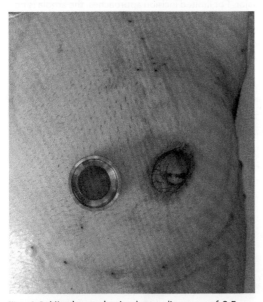

Fig. 6.9 Nipple-areola sized to a diameter of 2.5 cm, and marking for nipple reduction by wedge resection of the lower pole.

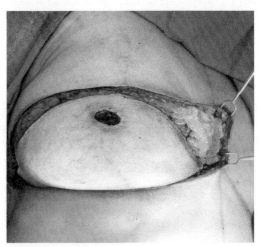

Fig. 6.12 Skin elevated at junction between breast parenchyma and subcutaneous fat.

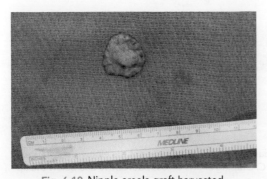

Fig. 6.10 Nipple-areola graft harvested.

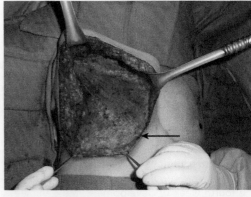

Fig. 6.13 Undermining of the inframammary crease. The arrow indicates the position of the inframammary crease.

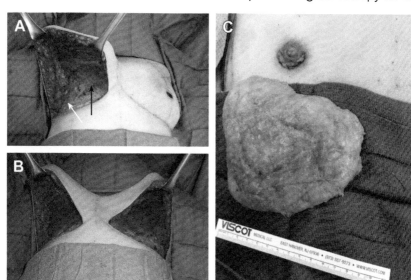

Fig. 6.14 (A) The breast is removed, and the pectoralis and serratus fascia are preserved. The white arrow indicates the serratus fascia, and the black arrow indicates the pectoralis fascia. The medial dissection stops at the sternal border; the lateral dissection proceeds over the serratus muscle, and the superior dissection stops at the clavicle. The axillary tail is removed, by either direct excision, liposuction, or a combination thereof. (B) Skin flaps elevated following bilateral, subcutaneous mastectomies. (C) Breast removed through limited incision mastectomy.

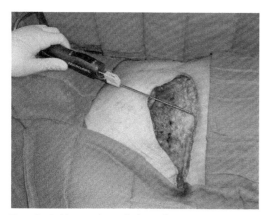

Fig. 6.15 Liposuction of the inframammary crease. Liposuction assists with discontiguous undermining of the inframammary crease.

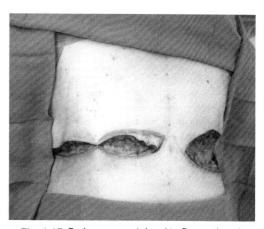

Fig. 6.17 Patient sat upright, skin flaps tailored.

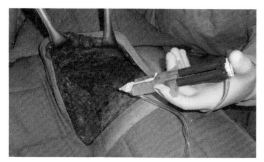

Fig. 6.16 Fibrin sealant placed in mastectomy cavity.

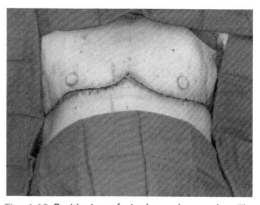

Fig. 6.18 Positioning of nipple-areola complex. The patient is sat upright, and the nipple-areola complex is positioned medial to the lateral border of the pectoralis major muscle and 1 to 2 cm above the inferior insertion of the pectoralis major muscle.

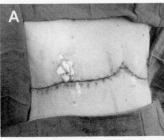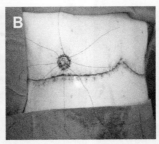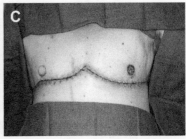

Fig. 6.19 (A) The planned site of the areola is de-epithelialized. (B) Fixation of nipple-areola graft. The nipple-areola graft is sutured in place, including the placement of quilting sutures. (C) Bolster dressing placed. The nipple-areola graft is dressed with petrolatum gauze soaked in bacitracin ointment and mineral oil. The bolster dressing is typically removed on postoperative day 4 or 5.

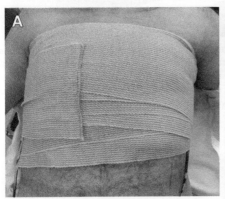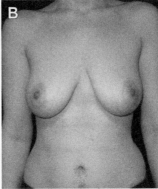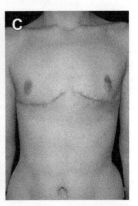

Fig. 6.20 (A) Postoperative chest dressing with elastic compression wrap and closed suction drains. (B) Preoperative photograph of patient undergoing chest surgery. (C) Postoperative photograph following double-incision chest surgery with free nipple-areola grafts, liposuction of chest, nipple and areola reduction, and areola repositioning.

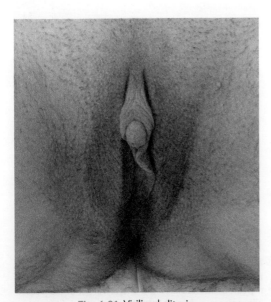

Fig. 6.21 Virilized clitoris.

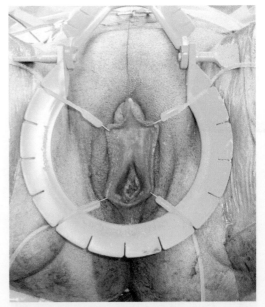

Fig. 6.22 Lone star retractor aids with exposure of ure-thra, clitoris, labia minora, and vagina.

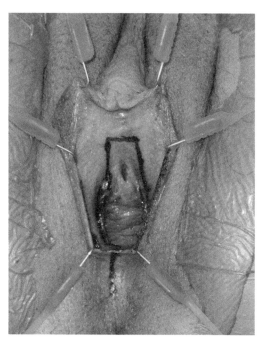

Fig. 6.23 Preoperative markings for creation of rectangular-shaped vestibular lining flap. This incision will also provide access for resection of the ventral chordee. The flap extends approximately one-third of the distance between the urethral orifice and the clitoris. A vaginal musculomucosal flap will be elevated and sutured to the vestibular lining flap, creating the proximal urethra.

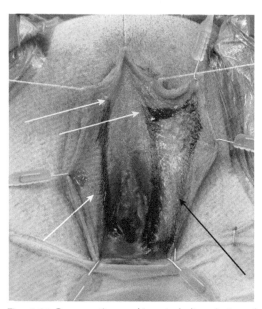

Fig. 6.24 Preoperative markings including design of the left labia minora flap and the contralateral right labia minora flap. The parallel incisions forming the rectangular vestibular lining flap are extended to the clitoris, demonstrated by the yellow arrows, and represent the medial incisions for the left and right labia minora flaps. The left flap, indicated by the black arrow, will form the ventral urethra, and the contralateral right flap, indicated by the right arrow, will be transposed over the left flap, providing a layered closure as well as the skin of the ventral penile shaft.

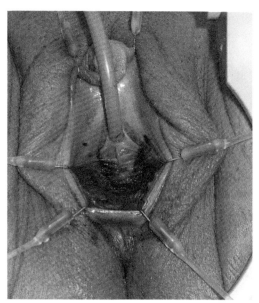

Fig. 6.25 Markings for the vaginal lining flap. The markings for the vaginal flap represent intravaginal extensions of the incisions used to create the rectangular lining flap.

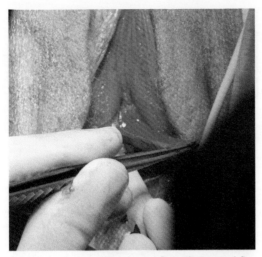

Fig. 6.26 Harvest of the vaginal flap. The vaginal flap will be sutured to the vestibular lining flap. These 2 flaps will form the proximal urethra.

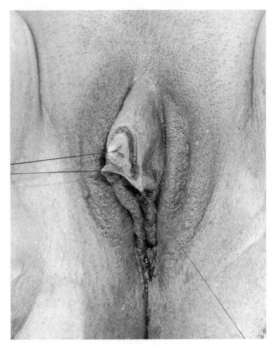

Fig. 6.28 Incision located at the junction of the glans clitoris and the clitoral hood. This incision facilitates elevation of the labial skin and exposure of the dorsal corporal bodies.

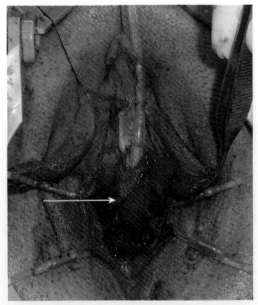

Fig. 6.27 Suture of the vaginal flap to the vestibular lining flap, forming the proximal urethra. The arrow indicates the proximal urethra. Note placement of the buccal mucosa graft on the underlying corporal bodies.

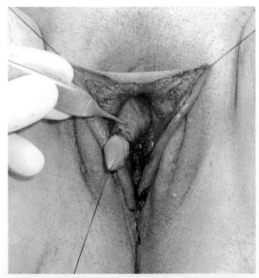

Fig. 6.29 Exposure of the clitoris. Note the position of the left dorsal neurovascular bundle, indicated by the forceps.

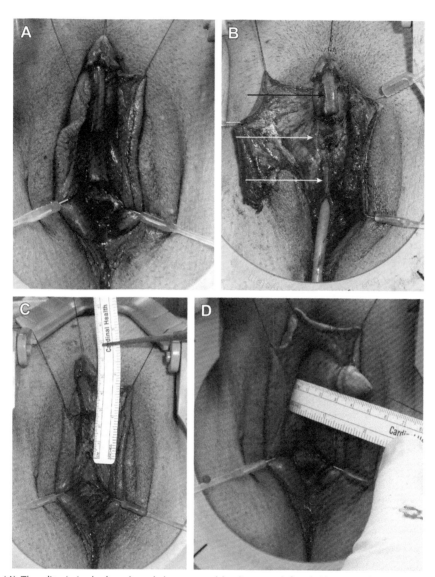

Fig. 6.30 (A) The clitoris is degloved, and the corporal bodies are defined. The ventral chordee has not been resected and tethers the clitoris. (B) Division of the ventral chordee. The division of the ventral chordee allows straightening and advancement of the clitoris. The white arrow indicates the vestibular lining flap. The yellow arrow indicates the defect created by division of the ventral chordee. The black arrow indicates the distal vestibular lining. (C and D) The clitoris straightened and lengthened. Clitoral lengthening is achieved with resection of the ventral chordee, and, when necessary, release of the suspensory ligament.

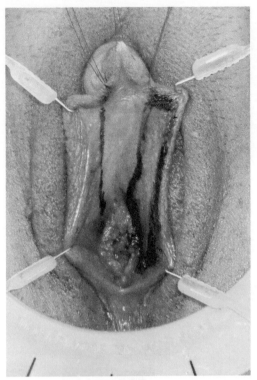

Fig. 6.31 Outline of bilateral labia minora flaps. The left labia minora flap is developed from the inner aspect of the left labia minora, and the right labia minora flap is developed from the contralateral side.

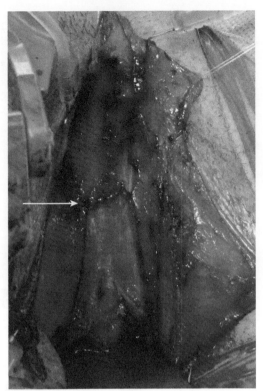

Fig. 6.33 Suture fixation of the vestibular flap to the corpora cavernosa. The arrow indicates the area of fixation.

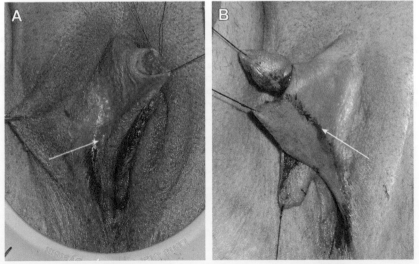

Fig. 6.32 (A) Outer, cutaneous surface of right labia minora remains intact. The right labia minora flap, indicated by arrow, will form the skin of the ventral penile shaft. (B) Outer, cutaneous surface of left labia minora flap, indicated by arrow, will be de-epithelialized. The left labia minora flap will form the ventral lining of the neourethra.

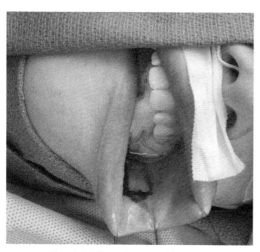

Fig. 6.34 Buccal mucosal harvest.

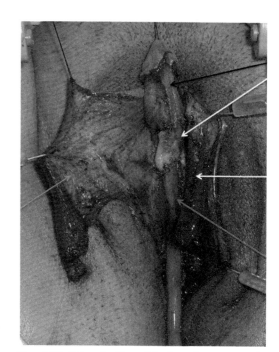

Fig. 6.36 Suture fixation of the buccal mucosa to the defect on ventral corporal bodies, created from resection of the ventral chordee. The red arrow indicates the vestibular line flap; the yellow arrow indicates the buccal mucosa graft; the black arrow indicates the distal vestibular lining; the white arrow indicates the left labia minora flap, and the green arrow indicates the right labia minora flap.

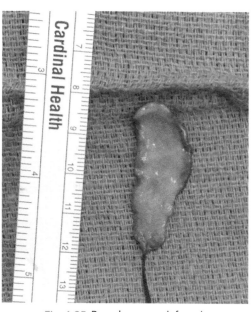

Fig. 6.35 Buccal mucosa defatted.

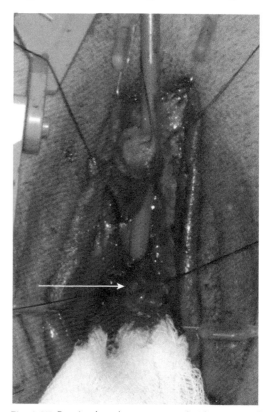

Fig. 6.37 Proximal urethra constructed with suturing of the vaginal flap to the vestibular lining flap, indicated by arrow.

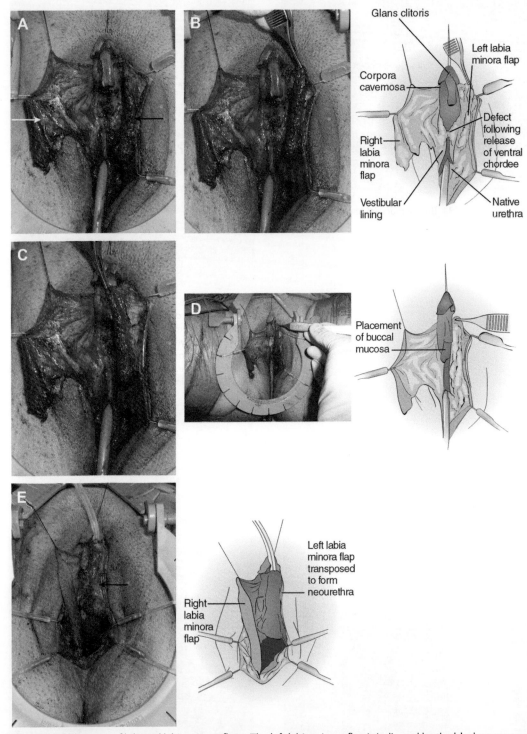

Fig. 6.38 (A) Elevation of bilateral labia minora flaps. The left labia minora flap is indicated by the black arrow, and the right labia minora flap is indicated by the white arrow. (B) Left labia minora flap transferred distally. (C) Left labia minora flap transposed. The left labia minora flap will form the ventral lining of the neourethra. (D) Left labia minora flap transposed (buccal mucosa in place). (E) Creation of ventral urethra. The pedicle of the left labia minora flap is indicated by the white arrow.

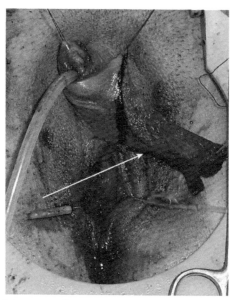

Fig. 6.39 Transposition of right labia minora flap over its left-sided counterpart. The 2 labia minora flaps create a layered closure over the urethra. The right-sided labia flap forms the ventral skin of the penile shaft. The redundant skin of the right labia minora, indicated by the white arrow, will be resected.

Fig. 6.40 Postoperative metoidioplasty.

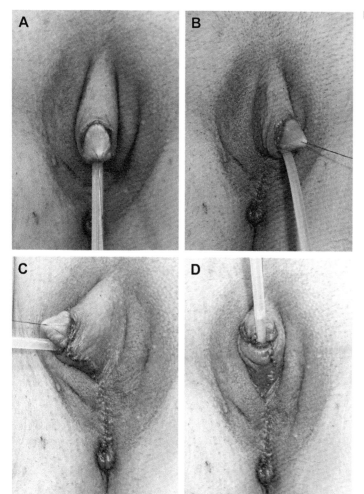

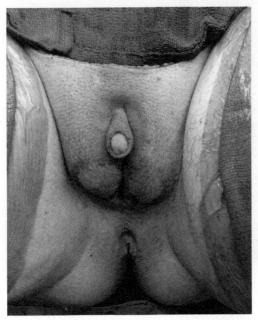

Fig. 6.41 Staged placement of testicular implants through Pfannenstiel incision. A mons resection is performed concurrent with the implant placement.

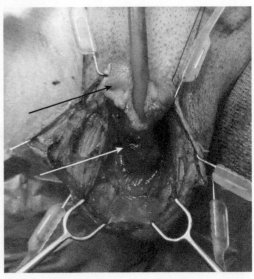

Fig. 6.44 Isolation of the urethra. The black arrow indicates the glans penis (former glans clitoris), and the white arrow indicates the urethra (of the former metoidioplasty). This portion of the urethra will form the new membranous urethra.

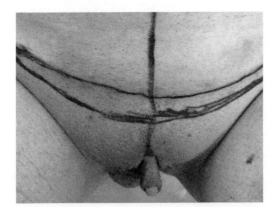

Fig. 6.42 Markings for mons resection. Scarpa fascia of the mons segment is anchored to the rectus sheath. Resection and repositioning of the mons gives the impression of a longer phallus.

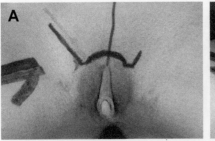

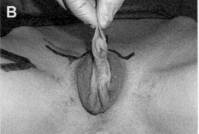

Fig. 6.43 Postoperative metoidioplasty in preparation for phalloplasty.

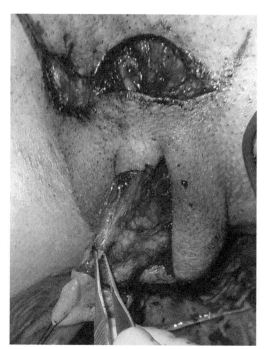

Fig. 6.45 Isolation of the left dorsal clitoral nerve. The left clitoral nerve is held by the forceps.

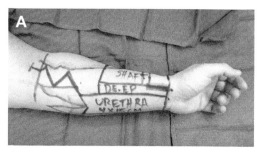
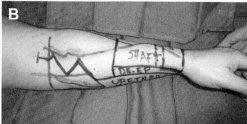
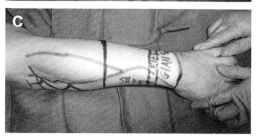

Fig. 6.46 Preoperative markings for radial forearm phalloplasty using a "tube-within-a-tube" technique. The ulnar border of the flap forms the penile urethra, and the volar and radial skin of the flap form the penile shaft. A central, intervening strip of skin between the urethra and shaft skin is excised and saved for later use in the glansplasty. Markings include the creation of the glans, which will be constructed from the distal portion of the forearm flap. The coronal ridge is formed using a distally based flap, located several centimeters proximal to the distal border of the forearm flap. The incision on the forearm is extended proximally in a zigzag fashion for access to the neurovascular structures.

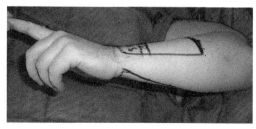

Fig. 6.47 Preoperative markings on the ulnar border of the forearm flap. Skin on the ulnar border of the forearm will remain in place. This skin will be drained by the basilic vein, which will remain in situ.

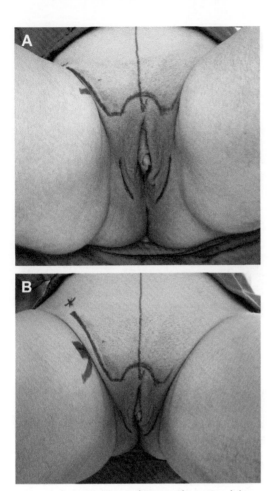

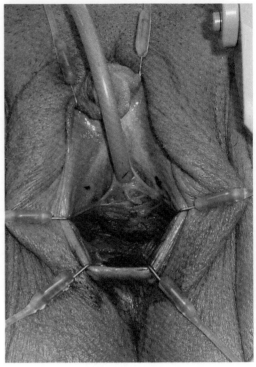

Fig. 6.49 Preparation for the vaginectomy.

Fig. 6.48 Preoperative markings on the perineal donor site. The omega-shaped donor site incision overlying the pubis, and the approximate locations of the ilioinguinal nerve and superficial femoral artery and vein and great saphenous vein are demonstrated. The incisions on the lateral aspect of the labia majora allow for medial transposition and construction of the scrotum.

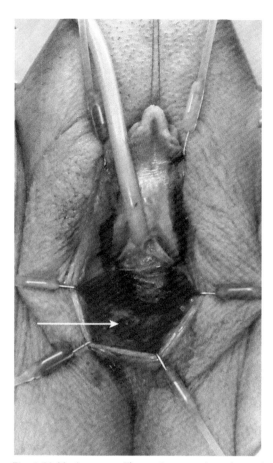

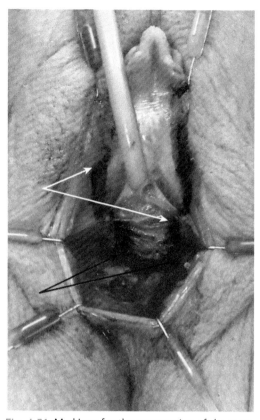

Fig. 6.51 Markings for the construction of the membranous urethra. The vestibular lining incisions, indicated by the white arrows, are marked between the native urethral meatus and the virilized clitoris. The markings for the vaginal flap, indicated by the black arrows, are contiguous with those of the vestibular lining flap.

Fig. 6.50 Vaginectomy. The vaginectomy is performed by removal of the vaginal epithelium, indicated by the arrow. The muscular layer of the vaginal wall is left intact. The anterior vaginal wall flap, used for construction of the proximal neourethra, is marked and left intact.

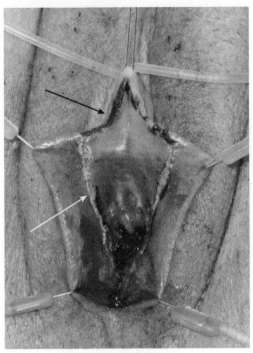

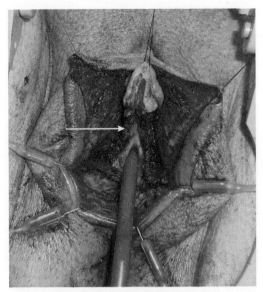

Fig. 6.54 Vestibular incisions, indicated by arrow, allow exposure of the lateral surface of the corporal bodies.

Fig. 6.52 Incisions on the vestibular lining. The vestibular lining will be tubularized to construct the membranous urethra. The white arrow indicates the portion of the vestibular lining that will be tubularized. The black arrow indicates the distal portion of the vestibular lining that will remain spatulated, to enlarge the distal os of the membranous urethra.

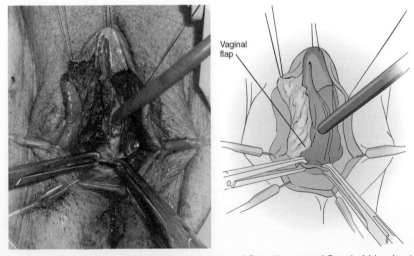

Fig. 6.53 Elevation of the anterior wall vaginal musculomucosal flap. The vaginal flap, held by the Allis clamps, is based distally at the urethral meatus.

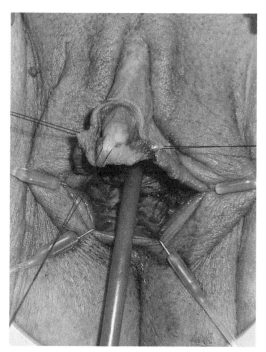

Fig. 6.55 Incision at the junction of the glans and the clitoral hood allows exposure of the dorsal corporal bodies.

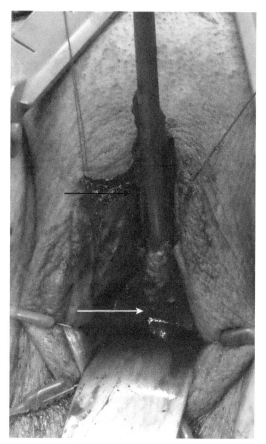

Fig. 6.56 Construction of the membranous urethra. The vestibular incisions, indicated by black arrow, are complete and contiguous with the vaginal wall flap, indicated by white arrow, and the clitoris is degloved.

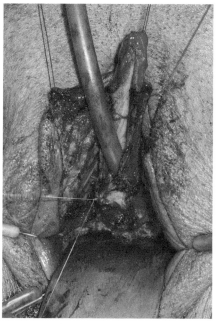

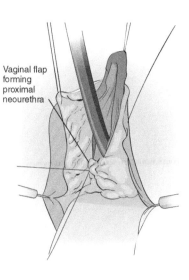

Vaginal flap forming proximal neourethra

Fig. 6.57 Construction of the proximal urethra. The proximal urethra is constructed with suturing of the vaginal wall flap to the vestibular lining.

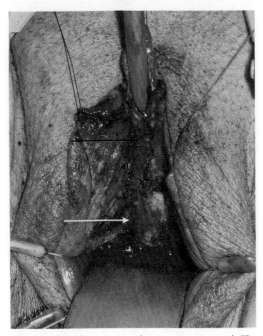

Fig. 6.58 Membranous urethra is reconstructed. The vestibular lining is tubularized over an 18-French catheter and indicated by the black arrow. The white arrow indicates the proximal urethra, constructed with the vaginal lining flap.

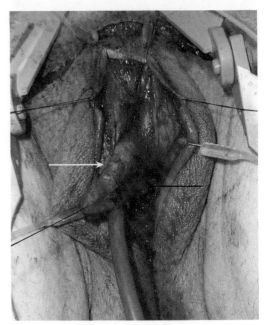

Fig. 6.60 Elevation of the labia minora and exposure of the clitoris and corporal bodies. The skin of the labia minora is elevated to the pubic symphysis. The glans clitoris has been de-epithelialized, and the left dorsal clitoral neurovascular bundle will be harvested for subsequent neurorrhaphy. The white arrow indicates the corporal bodies. The black arrow indicates the tubularized vestibular lining, now representing the membranous urethra.

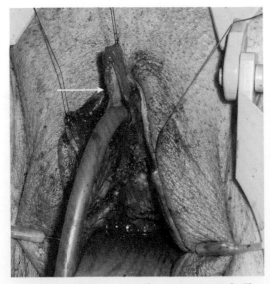

Fig. 6.59 Membranous urethra reconstructed. The distal os of the membranous urethra, indicated by the arrow, is spatulated, thereby widening the distal urethral anastomosis.

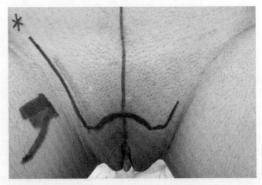

Fig. 6.61 Donor site incision in shape of an omega (Ω).

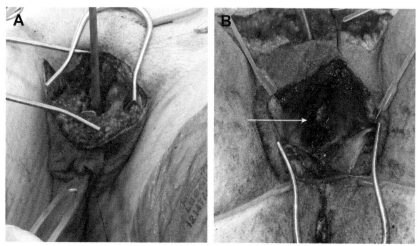

Fig. 6.62 (A) A subcutaneous tunnel is created between the perineum and the pubis. A retractor is placed in the subcutaneous tunnel, allowing passage of the clitoral-urethral construct into position at the pubic symphysis. (B) The clitoral-urethral construct is transferred subcutaneously. The arrow indicates the membranous urethra.

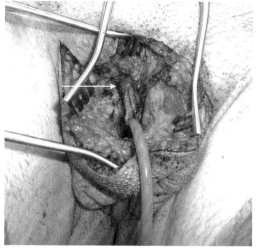

Fig. 6.63 Fixation of the de-epithelialized clitoris, indicated by the arrow, to the pubic symphysis. Fixation to the pubis stabilizes the clitoral-urethral construct.

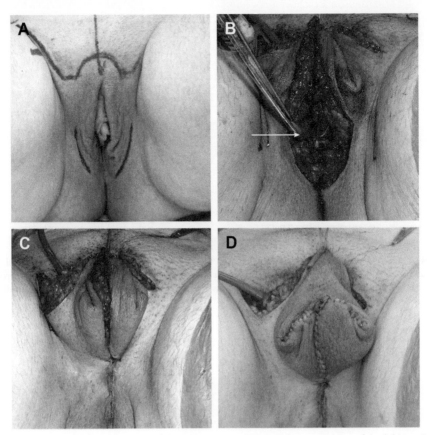

Fig. 6.64 (*A*) Incisions on the lateral border of the labia majora. (*B*) Medial transposition of the labia majora flaps. In addition, reconstruction of the pelvic floor is performed by layered closure of the superficial perineal muscles, indicated by the arrow, over the reconstructed membranous urethra. (*C*) Layered closure of the scrotum. (*D*) Scrotoplasty. The reconstructed scrotum is brought in position anterior to the legs.

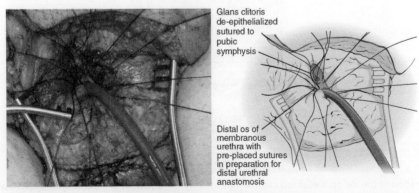

Glans clitoris de-epithelialized sutured to pubic symphysis

Distal os of membranous urethra with pre-placed sutures in preparation for distal urethral anastomosis

Fig. 6.65 Preplaced urethral sutures.

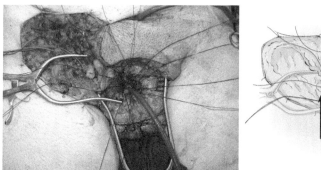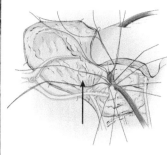

Fig. 6.66 Exposure of the recipient vessels with an oblique extension of the donor site incision. The incision for exposure of the femoral vessels parallels the inguinal ligament. The neurovascular pedicle of the forearm flap will be placed along the course from the pubic symphysis (position of phallus) to the femoral vessels. The arrow indicates the site along which the pedicle will be placed. Vessel loops encircle the superficial femoral artery.

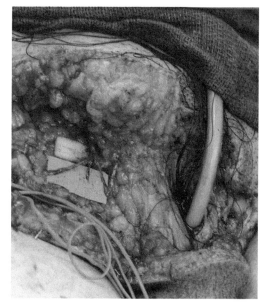

Fig. 6.67 The ilioinguinal nerve is exposed and divided distally for later coaptation to the lateral antebrachial cutaneous nerve.

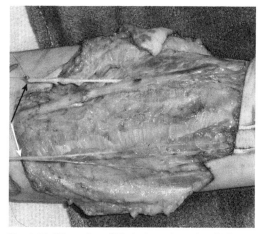

Fig. 6.68 Dissection of (1) the lateral antebrachial cutaneous nerve, indicated by the black arrow, adjacent to cephalic vein, and (2) the medial antebrachial cutaneous nerve, indicated by the white arrow, adjacent to the median antebrachial vein.

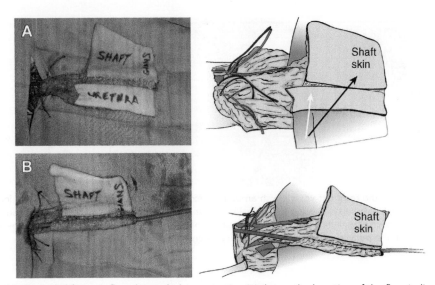

Fig. 6.69 (*A*) The radial forearm flap elevated, demonstrating (1) the urethral portion of the flap, indicated by the white arrow, and (2) the shaft portion of the flap, indicated by the black arrow. The intervening segment of skin, between the urethral and shaft portions of the flap, is excised and saved for later use in the glansplasty. (*B*) Tubularization and layered closure of the penile urethra over a catheter.

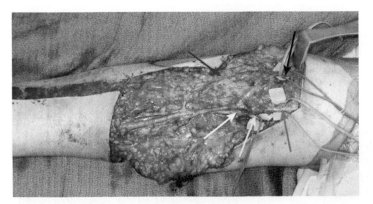

Fig. 6.70 Dissection of the neurovascular pedicle. Dissection includes: (1) cephalic vein (*green arrow*), (2) median antebrachial vein (*blue arrow*), (3) lateral antebrachial cutaneous nerve (*yellow arrow*), (4) medial antebrachial cutaneous nerve (*black arrow*), and (5) perforating branch (*white arrow*) communicating the deep and superficial venous systems.

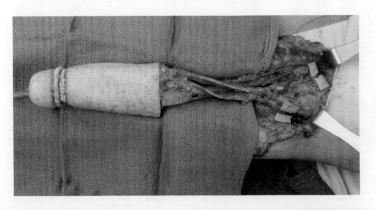

Fig. 6.71 Flap shaped in situ; neurovascular pedicle dissected.

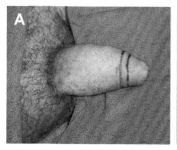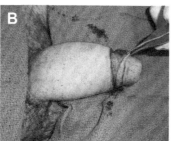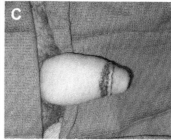

Fig. 6.72 (*A*) Markings for glansplasty. In this case, the glansplasty was performed 2 weeks following the phalloplasty. (*B*) Glansplasty and formation of the coronal ridge with elevation of the distally based flap. (*C*) Construction of coronal ridge and placement of skin graft at donor site of distally based flap.

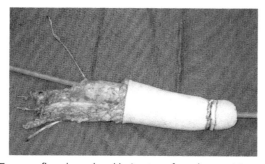

Fig. 6.73 Forearm flap shaped and being transferred to position at the pubis.

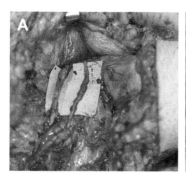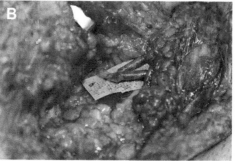

Fig. 6.74 Neurorrhaphies and placement of the nerve wraps.

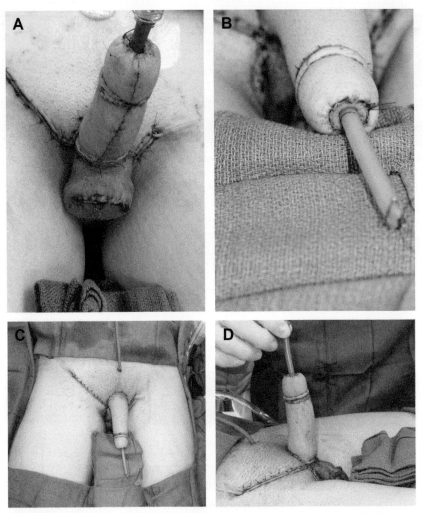

Fig. 6.75 (*A*) Phalloplasty with urethral lengthening, glansplasty, and scrotoplasty. (*B*) Urethral meatus. (*C, D*) Post-operative phalloplasty.

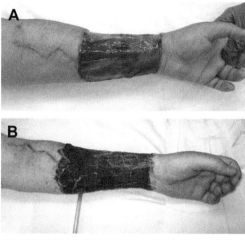

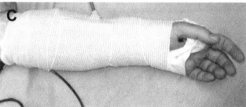

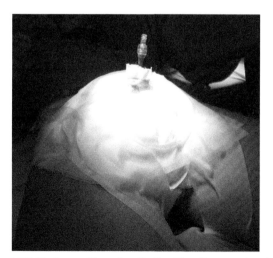

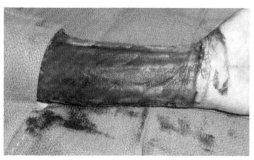

Fig. 6.78 Appearance of wound matrix, before skin graft, following removal of silicone bilayer.

Fig. 6.76 (A) Placement of bilayer wound matrix on the forearm donor site. (B) NPWT used to dress forearm donor site. (C) Light compression wrap applied to the forearm donor site.

Fig. 6.77 Phallus positioned vertically with soft gauze dressing.

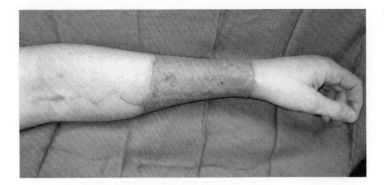

Fig. 6.79 Postoperative forearm donor site.

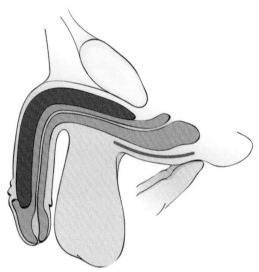

Fig. 6.80 Technique of "urethral milking." Unlike the natal male, in the phalloplasty patient, the bulbospongiosus muscle does not encircle the corpus spongiosum. As such, manual assistance ("urethral milking") may be required for expulsion of the last drops of urine.

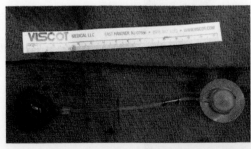

Fig. 6.81 Tissue expander used to enlarge the scrotal sac, before placement of the testicular implants.

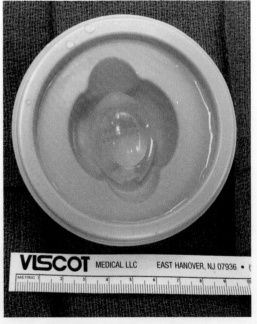

Fig. 6.82 Testicular prosthesis.

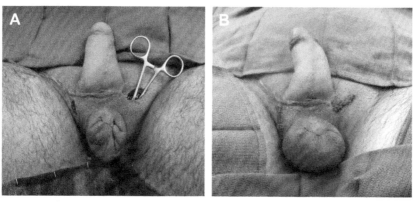

Fig. 6.83 (A) Insertion of testicular prostheses. Testicular prostheses inserted through previous phalloplasty donor site incision. (B) Testicular implants placed.

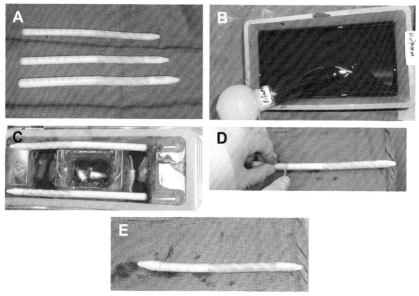

Fig. 6.84 (A) Malleable erectile prosthesis. Diameters: 9.5 mm, 11 mm, and 13 mm. (B and C) Antibiotic solution and device soaked in antibiotic solution. (D) Device cut to size. (E) Tip placed.

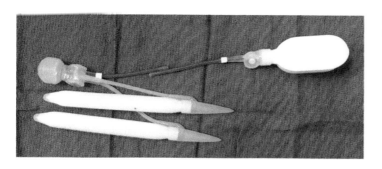

Fig. 6.85 Three-piece, dual-rod erectile prosthesis.

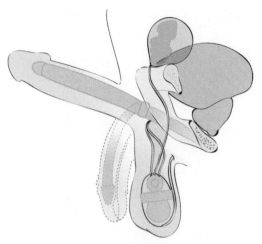

Fig. 6.86 Placement of inflatable erectile prosthesis. The pump is placed in the scrotum, and the reservoir is placed in the retroperitoneal position.

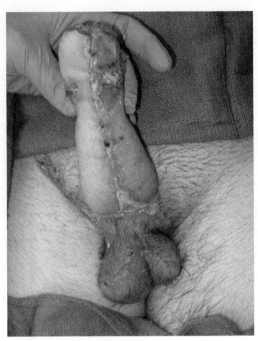

Fig. 6.88 Delayed wound healing in radial forearm phalloplasty.

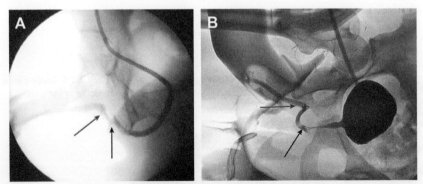

Fig. 6.87 (A, B) Post-phalloplasty cystogram. The 2 urethral anastomoses are demonstrated: (1) the black arrow demonstrates the proximal urethral anastomosis between the native urethra and the membranous urethra, and (2) the red arrow demonstrates the distal anastomosis between the membranous urethra and the penile urethra.

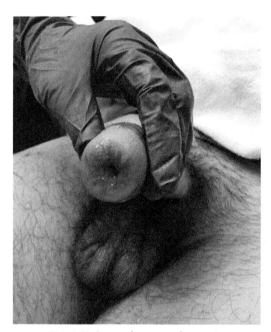

Fig. 6.89 Incomplete meatal stenosis.

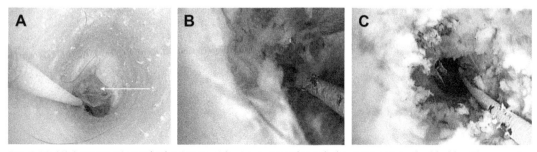

Fig. 6.90 (A) Anastomotic urethral stricture with wire passing through the stricture into the bladder. The arrow indicates the location of the stricture. (B) Direct visual internal urethrotomy using laser. An anastomotic urethral stricture undergoing Holmium laser urethrotomy. (C) Anastomotic urethral stricture with wire passing through the stricture after Holmium laser urethrotomy.

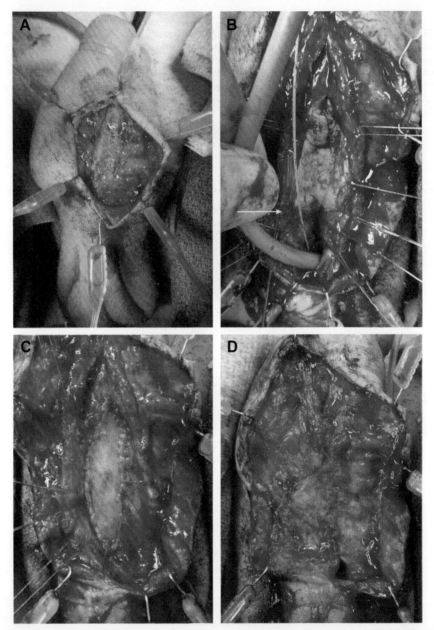

Fig. 6.91 (A) Incision in the pendulous urethra for exposure of a urethral stricture. (B) Incised urethra at the site of stricture. Stay sutures are placed at the lateral edges of the urethral plate to aid with exposure. The white arrow indicates the stricture at the distal anastomosis. The distal anastomosis is between the membranous urethra and penile urethra. (C) Placement of buccal mucosa graft on the ventral urethra. (D) Closure of the periurethral tissue.

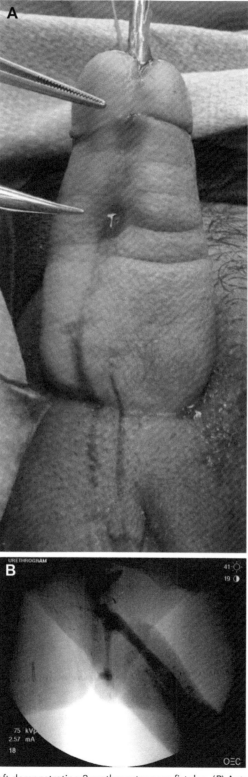

Fig. 6.92 (A) Ventral penile shaft demonstrating 2 urethrocutaneous fistulae. (B) Anterograde urethrogram demonstrating a urethrocutaneous fistula.

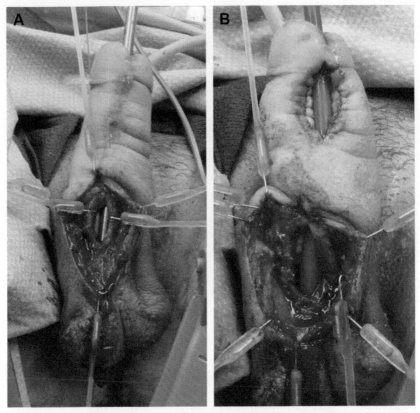

Fig. 6.93 (*A*) Excision of one of the fistulae tracts. (*B*) Staged fistula repair with placement of a buccal mucosa graft.

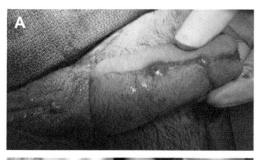

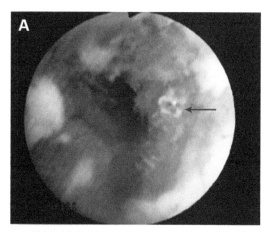

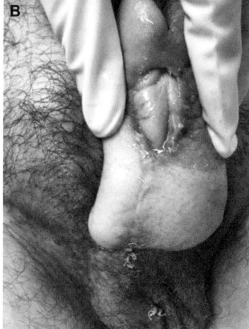

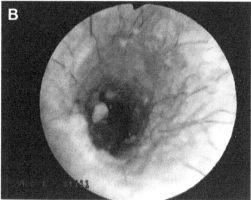

Fig. 6.95 (A) Urethroscopy images demonstrating persistent, nonabsorbable suture, indicated by red arrow, 6 months after surgery. (B) Urethroscopy images demonstrating hair in the urethra.

Fig. 6.94 (A) Ventral penile shaft demonstrating a urethrocutaneous fistula. (B) Two-stage urethroplasty for repair of a urethrocutaneous fistula.

REFERENCES

1. Monstrey S, Selvaggi G, Ceulemans P, et al. Chest-wall contouring surgery in female-to-male transsexuals: a new algorithm. Plast Reconstr Surg 2008;121(3):849–59.
2. Hage JJ, van Turnhout AA. Long-term outcome of metaidoioplasty in 70 female-to-male transsexuals. Ann Plast Surg 2006;57(3):312–6.
3. Hage JJ. Metaidoioplasty: an alternative phalloplasty technique in transsexuals. Plast Reconstr Surg 1996;97(1):161–7.
4. Hage JJ, van Turnhout AA, Dekker JJ, et al. Saving labium minus skin to treat possible urethral stenosis in female-to-male transsexuals. Ann Plast Surg 2006;56(4):456–9.
5. Djordjevic ML, Bizic M, Stanojevic D, et al. Urethral lengthening in metoidioplasty (female-to-male sex reassignment surgery) by combined buccal mucosa graft and labia minora flap. Urology 2009;74(2):349–53.
6. Hoebeke P, Selvaggi G, Ceulemans P, et al. Impact of sex reassignment surgery on lower urinary tract function. Eur Urol 2005;47(3):398–402.
7. Vyas JB, Ganpule AP, Muthu V, et al. Balloon dilatation for male urethral strictures "revisited". Urol Ann 2013;5(4):245–8.
8. Jackson MJ, Veeratterapillay R, Harding CK, et al. Intermittent self-dilatation for urethral stricture disease in males. Cochrane Database Syst Rev 2014;(12):CD010258.
9. Jain SK, Kaza RC, Singh BK. Evaluation of holmium laser versus cold knife in optical internal urethrotomy for the management of short segment urethral stricture. Urol Ann 2014;6(4):328–33.
10. Pansadoro V, Emiliozzi P. Internal urethrotomy in the management of anterior urethral strictures: long-term followup. J Urol 1996;156(1):73–5.
11. Somerville JJ, Adeyemi OA, Clark PB. Long-term results of two-stage urethroplasty. Br J Urol 1985;57(6):742–5.

CHAPTER 7

Conclusion

Although some states and/or countries no longer require surgery for change of legal status, others do. In such cases, following surgery, an individual may request a letter addressed to the relevant governmental agencies petitioning for a change of legal "sex." This letter may be important for the individual's legal documents (ie, driver's license, passport, social security) and should include the nature of the treatment rendered. Individual state laws may vary in regard to the requirements for change of legal documents (Fig. 7.1).

This text provides a basis for understanding the principles of transgender surgery. For many surgeons, this will be their first exposure to these procedures. This book, in conjunction with ongoing educational offerings, will help build a foundation upon which surgeons may gain exposure to the field of gender confirming procedures.

It must be emphasized and understood that continued collaboration between the surgeon, mental health professional, and medical physician is important in providing comprehensive care to transgender individuals. In addition, continued research focused on objective parameters and reporting of outcomes data will foster innovation and continued improvements in surgical techniques.

(insert date)

Loren S. Schechter MD, FACS
9000 Waukegan Road
Suite 210
Morton Grove, IL 60053

Illinois State License Number:
DEA License Number:

To Whom It May Concern:

This letter is in reference to (insert name) date of birth (insert), and outlines (his/her/their)
surgical procedure (s). On (insert date), (insert name) underwent gender confirmation surgery at
(insert hospital). This procedure involved: (select procedure)

(vaginoplasty (creation of vaginal canal), orchiectomy (removal of testicles), penectomy
(removal of the penis), labiaplasty (creation of labia minora), clitoroplasty (creation of clitoris),
and urethroplasty (restoration of urethra))

(phalloplasty (creation of a penis), scrotoplasty (creation of a scrotum), vaginectomy (removal of
vagina), and colpocleisis (closure of the vagina).

(metoidioplasty (lengthening of the clitoris), scrotoplasty (creation of a scrotum), vaginectomy
(removal of vagina), and colpocleisis (closure of vagina).

(chest surgery (bilateral mastectomies).

(insert name) has been in compliance with the guidelines outlined by the World Professional
Association for Transgender Health and has had the appropriate clinical treatment for gender
transition to the new (male/female) status.

I declare under penalty of perjury under the laws of the United States that the forgoing is true and
correct.

If you have any questions or concerns, please do not hesitate to contact me.

Sincerely,

Loren S. Schechter, MD, FACS

Fig. 7.1 Letter for change of legal status.

Appendices

Adapted from the American Society of Plastic Surgeons Informed Consent product.

APPENDIX A: VAGINOPLASTY CONSENT

Informed consent—agreement for male-to-female gender confirmation surgery (vaginoplasty, clitoroplasty, labiaplasty, penectomy, bilateral orchiectomy, urethroplasty, possible skin grafts)

Instructions

This informed consent document has been prepared to inform you of male-to-female gender confirmation surgery, its risks, as well as alternative treatments. It is important that you read this information carefully and completely. Please initial each page, indicating that you have read the page, and sign the consent for surgery as proposed by Loren S. Schechter, MD.

Informed consent documents are used to communicate information about the proposed surgical treatment of a disease or condition along with disclosure of risks and alternative forms of treatment(s). The informed consent process defines principles of risk disclosure that should generally meet the needs of most patients in most circumstances.

However, informed consent documents should not be considered all inclusive in defining other methods of care and risks encountered. Informed consent documents are not intended to define or serve as the standard of medical care. Standards of medical care are determined on the basis of all of the facts involved in an individual case and are subject to changes as scientific knowledge and technology advance and as practice patterns evolve.

Introduction

Male-to-female gender confirmation surgery is a surgical procedure to transform male anatomy into female anatomy. This surgery involves a total penectomy (removal of the penis), bilateral orchiectomy (removal of both testicles), construction of a vagina from the penile skin and/or with scrotal skin and/or a skin graft, construction of a clitoris, labiaplasty, and creation of a new urethral opening.

Alternative Treatments

Alternative forms of care consist of not undergoing surgery. Alternative types of surgery involve the creation of a vagina using pieces of the intestine (for example, sigmoid colon) or skin from elsewhere on the body such as the thighs or abdomen. Risks and potential complications are associated with alternative forms of treatment that involve surgery.

1. I,_____, hereby authorize Loren S. Schechter, MD and such assistants and/or designees as may be selected to perform any or all of the following operations intended to transform male anatomy into female anatomy: total penectomy (removal of the penis), bilateral orchiectomy (removal of both testicles), construction of a vagina from the penile skin and/or with scrotal skin and/or a skin graft, a clitoris, labiaplasty, and creation of a new urethral opening.

2. This operation has been explained to me by Dr Loren S. Schechter, and I understand the nature and consequences of the procedure. I understand that during the course of the operation and/or medical treatment, unforeseen conditions could become apparent that may necessitate an extension of the original procedures or different procedures than those set forth above. I therefore authorize and request that Dr Loren S. Schechter and his assistants and/or designees perform such surgical procedures or render such medical treatments as are necessary and desirable in the exercise of professional judgment. The authority granted under this paragraph shall extend to treating the conditions that are both known and unknown to Dr Schechter at the time the operation is begun.

I also understand that it is impossible for a surgeon to disclose every conceivable risk, however remote. Although good results are expected, complications cannot be anticipated; therefore, there can be no guarantee either expressed or implied, as to the result of this surgery because the practice of medicine is not an exact science. Every surgical procedure involves a certain amount of risk, and it is important that you understand the risks involved with male-to-female gender reassignment surgery. Although most patients do not experience the following complications, you should discuss each of them with Dr Schechter to make sure that you understand the possible consequences of male-to-female gender reassignment surgery. The following points have been made specifically clear and are intended to provide information:

A. Scars result from any surgical procedure, but efforts are made to conceal or make them as inconspicuous as possible. Excessive scarring can occur. In rare cases, abnormal scars may result. Scars may be unattractive and of different color than the surrounding skin. Additional treatments including surgery may be necessary to treat abnormal scarring.

B. Signs of inflammation such as tenderness, swelling, and discoloration (redness or black and blueness) occur that may last for several weeks or until the wound is completely healed. Residual swelling and redness can last a year or more.

C. Skin sensation: Numbness in or around the operative site may occur and may persist for an indefinite period of time. Occasionally this may be permanent. Numbness may also occur in the hands, arms, or legs due to the position of the body during surgery. This may or may not be permanent.

D. Infection may occur. Should an infection occur, treatment including antibiotics or additional surgery may be necessary.

E. Bleeding is possible during or after surgery. Should postoperative bleeding occur, it may require emergency treatment to drain accumulated blood (hematoma) or blood transfusion. I consent to the administration of whole blood or blood components. It has been explained to me that there is the possibility of ill effects including, but not limited to, infection and other diseases resulting from the administration of blood or blood components. I acknowledge and agree that neither the doctor nor the Hospital provides any guarantee nor warranty with respect to the blood or blood components. Should blood transfusion be required—you will be responsible for this additional cost.

F. Delayed healing: Wound disruption or delayed wound healing is possible. Some areas may not heal normally and/or may take a long time to heal. Some areas of the skin may die. This may require frequent dressing changes or further surgery to remove the nonhealed tissue. Unintentional interruption of blood supply to a flap, skin graft, or part of the operated area may result in its loss. Smokers have a greater risk of skin loss and wound-healing complications.

G. Seroma: Fluid accumulations infrequently occur. Should this problem occur, it may require additional procedures for drainage of fluid.

H. Asymmetry (noticeable difference in the size and shape) between the 2 sides of the operated area may result when both right and left sides are operated upon.

I. Rectal injury: Injury to the rectum may occur that could necessitate immediate closure of the opening; closure of whatever vagina has been created; and the immediate or later creation of a colostomy (exteriorization of the colon in order that waste does not pass through the rectum).

J. Urethral, bladder, intestinal injury: Injury to the urethra, urinary bladder, or peritoneal cavity is a possibility and could cause later scar contracture or other unforeseeable problems in the future, and/or require additional surgery.

K. Stenosis: Shortening of the newly made vagina may occur secondary to scar contracture deep within the vaginal vault.

L. Blood clots: Although rare, embolism from a blood clot may happen, which could result in death.

M. Allergic reactions: In rare cases, local allergies to tape, suture material, or topical preparations have been reported. Systemic reactions, which are more serious, may occur to drugs used during surgery and prescription medicines. Allergic reactions may require additional treatment.

N. Pain: Chronic pain may occur very infrequently from nerves becoming trapped in scar tissue.

O. Other: You may be disappointed with the results of surgery. Occasionally, it is necessary to perform additional surgery to improve your results. In addition, completely unpredictable and unusual complications, although extremely rare, including even death, may occur. I understand that because of the nature of the above procedures, it is impossible to predict all the possible psychiatric and physiologic results. Some of the possible complications explained to me that can be involved in these procedures include in addition to those set forth above but not by way of limitation, are the following: severe loss of blood, infection, cardiac arrest, poor cosmetic results, permanent pain and discomfort, adverse affects from anesthesia, and psychiatric disorders.

Additional Surgery Necessary

Should complications occur, additional surgery or other treatments may be necessary. Even though risks and complications occur infrequently, the risks cited are particularly associated with male-to-female gender confirmation surgery.

1. I understand this operation is totally irreversible and that I no longer will be able to have intercourse as a male or to conceive children. I also understand that Dr Loren S. Schechter does not guarantee any sexual pleasure or function as a result of the above stated procedures.

2. I consent to the administration of such anesthetics as may be considered necessary or advisable by the physician or anesthetist responsible for this service. There is the possibility of complications, injury, and even death from all forms of surgical anesthesia or sedation.

3. I consent to be photographed before, during, and after treatment, and I understand that these photographs are the visual part of my clinical record and are the property of Dr Loren S. Schechter and may be published in scientific journals and/or shown for professional reasons. I hereby authorize Dr Loren S. Schechter and his assistants and/or his designees to use preoperative, intraoperative, and postoperative photographs, videotapes, and/or voice recordings for professional medical purposes deemed appropriate, including, but not limited to, showing these images on public or commercial television, electronic digital networks, for purposes of medical education, patient education, lay publication, or during lectures to medical or lay groups. I understand that I will not be entitled to monetary payment or any other consideration as a result of any use of these images and/or my interview. I waive any right or option to inspect or approve the finished product or advertising or other copy that may be used along with the photographs, videotape, and voice recordings. I hereby grant Dr Loren S. Schechter the unlimited right to use such photographs, videotapes, and/or voice recordings as he deems appropriate, at his sole discretion.

4. For purposes of advancing medical education, I consent to the admittance of observers in the operating room. I have been advised, and I agree, that the surgical operation may be performed by a team of doctors, including one or more attending doctors, residents, and medical students.

5. I consent to additional practitioners performing the procedure, or important aspects of the procedure, different from those now contemplated, whether or not arising from presently unforeseen conditions, whom Dr Schechter and/or his assistants and/or designees may consider necessary or advisable in the course of this operation.

6. I consent to the disposal of any tissue, medical devices, or body parts that may be removed.

7. I have been informed by Dr Loren S. Schechter that there are separate fees for surgical, medical, psychological, and anesthesia services, as well as hospital fees. Additional costs may occur should complications develop from the surgery. Charges for secondary surgery or revisionary surgery would be your responsibility.

8. I certify that I have read and fully understand the above consent and agreement, which has been preceded by explanations by Dr Loren S. Schechter. I also certify that I have read and understand Dr Schechter's standard form letter regarding Gender Confirmation Surgery. His explanations in no way vary from the contents of this consent statement or his form letter and are understood by me. I agree not to revoke, limit, or alter this consent.

I fully understand all of the above, and I am satisfied with the explanation. I have no further questions. It has been explained to me in a way that I understand the treatment to be undertaken, the alternative methods of treatment, and the risks to the treatment. I authorize Loren S. Schechter, MD and his assistants and/or designees to perform any or all of the procedures discussed in this male-to-female gender reassignment surgery consent.

Patient_____

Date_____

Witness_____

In order to signify that you have read and understood the male-to-female gender confirmation surgery consent form, please complete the questionnaire.

Please list 3 possible complications of surgery:

1. _____

2. _____

3. _____

Please write in your own handwriting, "I have read and understood the male-to-female gender confirmation surgery consent form, and all of my questions have been fully answered" in the space provided below.

_____

_____

_____

_____

_____

Complete the following sentence found within the consent form:

"Should complications occur, _____."

Patient_____

Date_____

Witness_____

APPENDIX B: CHEST SURGERY CONSENT

Informed consent—mastectomy (chest surgery, possible nipple graft, possible liposuction) for gender confirmation

Instructions

This is an informed-consent document that has been prepared to help Dr Schechter inform you about mastectomy (chest surgery, possible nipple graft, possible liposuction) for gender confirmation, its risks, and alternative treatments.

It is important that you read this information carefully and completely. Please initial each page, indicating that you have read the page, and sign the consent for surgery as proposed by your plastic surgeon.

General Information

Mastectomy (chest surgery, possible nipple graft, possible liposuction) for gender confirmation is a part of the female-to-male gender confirmation process. The best candidates are those who understand the procedure and have realistic expectations about the results. This surgery involves removal of the female breast gland, removal of excess breast skin when necessary, repositioning of the nipple and areola as a free graft when necessary, and liposuction when necessary. There are both risks and complications associated with alternative surgical forms of treatment.

Alternative Treatment

Mastectomy (chest surgery, possible nipple graft, possible liposuction) for gender confirmation is an elective surgical operation. Alternative treatment would consist of not undergoing surgery, and in select patients, liposuction alone has been used to reduce the size of breasts. Potential risks and complications are associated with alternative techniques that involve surgery.

Risks of Mastectomy (Chest Surgery, Possible Nipple Graft, Possible Liposuction) Surgery

Every surgical procedure involves a certain amount of risk, and it is important that you understand the risks involved with *Mastectomy (chest surgery, possible nipple graft, possible liposuction) for gender confirmation.* An individual's choice to undergo a surgical procedure is based on the comparison of the risk to potential benefit. Although most patients do not experience these complications, you should discuss each of them with your plastic surgeon to make sure you understand the risks, potential complications, and consequences of mastectomy for gender confirmation.

Bleeding
It is possible, although unusual, to have problems with bleeding before, during, or after surgery. Should postoperative bleeding occur, it may require emergency treatment to stop the bleeding or remove an accumulation of blood (hematoma). It may require a blood transfusion. Do not take any aspirin or anti-inflammatory medications for 7 days before surgery, because this contributes to a greater risk of bleeding. Nonprescription "herbs" and dietary supplements can increase the risk of surgical bleeding. Hematoma can occur at any time following injury to the breast.

Infection
Infection is unusual after this type of surgery. It may appear in the immediate postoperative period or at any time following the surgery. Subacute or chronic infections may be difficult to diagnose. Should an infection occur, treatment including antibiotics or additional surgery may be necessary. Individuals with a weakened immune system (currently receiving chemotherapy or drugs to suppress the immune system) may be at greater risk for infection.

Change in nipple sensation and skin sensation
If a free nipple graft is performed, there will be no nipple sensation after surgery. After several months or years, some patients will regain partial sensation. Partial or permanent loss of nipple and skin sensation in one or both nipples may occur after surgery even if nipple grafts are not performed. Changes in sensation may affect sexual response.

Skin scarring
Although good wound healing after a surgical procedure is expected, abnormal scars may occur within both the skin and deeper tissues. Scars may be unattractive and of different color than surrounding skin tone. There is the possibility of visible marks from sutures used for wound closure. Additional treatments may be needed to treat abnormal scarring after surgery.

Unsatisfactory result
You may be disappointed with the results of surgery. Asymmetry in nipple location and unanticipated chest wall shape and size may occur after surgery. Unsatisfactory surgical scar location may occur. It may be necessary to perform additional surgery to improve your results.

Long-term results
Subsequent alterations in chest wall shape may occur as the result of aging, weight loss or gain, or other circumstances not related to the original mastectomy surgery. Skin sagging may naturally occur.

Pain
Abnormal scarring in skin and the deeper tissues of the chest may produce pain.

Firmness
Excessive firmness of the chest wall can occur after surgery due to internal scarring or fat necrosis. The occurrence of this is not predictable. If an area of fat necrosis or scarring appears, this may require biopsy or additional surgical treatment.

Delayed healing
Wound disruption or delayed wound healing is possible. Some areas of the breast and/or chest skin or nipple region may not heal normally and/or may take a long time to heal. It is even possible to have loss of skin or nipple tissue. This may require frequent dressing changes or further surgery to remove the nonliving tissue.

Smokers have a greater risk of skin loss and wound-healing complications

Asymmetry
Some breast asymmetry naturally occurs in most men and women. Differences in breast and nipple shape, size, or symmetry may also occur after surgery. Additional surgery may be necessary to revise asymmetry after a mastectomy for gender confirmation.

Breast cancer
Breast disease and breast cancer can occur independently of breast surgery, even after removal of breast tissue. It is recommended that all patients perform regular self-examination of their breasts, have

mammograms according to American Cancer Society guidelines, and seek professional care should a breast lump be detected.

Breast feeding

Because the breast glands are removed during surgery, breast feeding will not be possible after mastectomy for gender confirmation.

Surgical anesthesia

Both local and general anesthesia involve risk. There is the possibility of complications, injury, and even death from all forms of surgical anesthesia or sedation.

Allergic reactions

In rare cases, local allergies to tape, suture material, or topical preparations have been reported. Systemic reactions, which are more serious, may result from drugs used during surgery and prescription medications. Allergic reactions may require additional treatment.

Pulmonary complications

Pulmonary complications may occur secondarily to blood clots (pulmonary emboli) or partial collapse of the lungs after general anesthesia. Should either of these complications occur, you may require hospitalization and additional treatment. Pulmonary emboli can be life-threatening or fatal in some circumstances.

Additional Surgery Necessary

Should complications occur, additional surgery or other treatments may be necessary. Even though risks and complications occur infrequently, the risks cited are the ones that are particularly associated with mastectomy (chest surgery, possible nipple graft, possible liposuction) for gender confirmation. There are many variable conditions that may influence the long-term result of breast surgery. Secondary surgery may be necessary to perform additional tightening or repositioning of the nipples, areola, or chest skin. Other complications and risks can occur but are even more uncommon. The practice of medicine and surgery is not an exact science. Although good results are expected, there is no guarantee or warranty expressed or implied on the results that may be obtained.

Health Insurance

Mastectomy for gender confirmation may not be covered by your insurance. Please carefully review your health insurance subscriber-information pamphlet, call your insurance company, and discuss this further with your plastic surgeon. Many insurance plans exclude coverage for secondary or revisionary surgery.

Financial Responsibilities

The cost of surgery involves several charges for the services provided. This includes fees charged by your doctor, the cost of surgical supplies, laboratory tests, and possible outpatient hospital charges, depending on where the surgery is performed. Depending on whether the cost of surgery is covered by an insurance plan, you will be responsible for necessary copayments, deductibles, and charges not covered. Additional costs may occur should complications develop from the surgery. Secondary surgery or hospital day-surgery charges involved with revisionary surgery would also be your responsibility.

Disclaimer

Informed-consent documents are used to communicate information about the proposed surgical treatment of a disease or condition along with disclosure of risks and alternative forms of treatment(s). The informed-consent process attempts to define principles of risk disclosure that should generally meet the needs of most patients in most circumstances.

However, informed-consent documents should not be considered all inclusive in defining other methods of care and risks encountered. Your plastic surgeon may provide you with additional or different information, which is based on all the facts in your particular case and the state of medical knowledge.

Informed-consent documents are not intended to define or serve as the standard of medical care. Standards of medical care are determined on the basis of all the facts involved in an individual case and are subject to change as scientific knowledge and technology advance and as practice patterns evolve.

It is important that you read the above information carefully and have all of your questions answered before signing the consent on the next page.

Consent for Surgery/Procedure or Treatment

1. I hereby authorize Dr Loren Schechter and such assistants as may be selected to perform the following procedure or treatment:

I have read the following information sheet: Informed consent—mastectomy (chest surgery, possible nipple graft, possible liposuction) for gender confirmation.

2. I recognize that during the course of the operation and medical treatment or anesthesia, unforeseen conditions may necessitate different procedures than those above. I therefore authorize the above physician and assistants or designees to perform such other procedures that are in the exercise of his or her professional judgment necessary and desirable. The authority granted under this paragraph shall include all conditions that require treatment and are not known to my physician at the time the procedure is begun.

3. I consent to the administration of such anesthetics considered necessary or advisable. I understand that all forms of anesthesia involve risk and the possibility of complications, injury, and sometimes death.

4. I acknowledge that no guarantee has been given by anyone as to the results that may be obtained.

5. I consent to the photographing or televising of the operation(s) or procedure(s) to be performed, including appropriate portions of my body, for medical, scientific, or educational purposes, provided the pictures do not reveal my identity.

6. For purposes of advancing medical education, I consent to the admittance of observers to the operating room.

7. I consent to the disposal of any tissue, medical devices, or body parts that may be removed.

8. I authorize the release of my Social Security Number to appropriate agencies for legal reporting and medical-device registration, if applicable.

9. It has been explained to me in a way that I understand:

    a. The above treatment or procedure to be undertaken.

    b. There may be alternative procedures or methods of treatment.

    c. There are risks to the procedure or treatment proposed.

I fully understand all of the above, and I am satisfied with the explanation. I have no further questions. It has been explained to me in a way that I understand the treatment to be undertaken, the alternative methods of treatment, and the risks to the treatment. I authorize Loren S. Schechter, MD and his assistants and/or designees to perform any or all of the procedures discussed in this chest surgery consent.

Patient_____

Date_____

Witness_____

In order to signify that you have read and understood the chest surgery consent form, please complete the questionnaire.

Please list 3 possible complications of surgery:

1. _____

2. _____

3. _____

Please write in your own handwriting, "I have read and understood the chest surgery consent form, and all of my questions have been fully answered" in the space provided below.

_____

_____

_____

_____

_____

Complete the following sentence found within the consent form:

"Should complications occur, _____."

Patient_____

Date_____

Witness_____

I CONSENT TO THE TREATMENT OR PROCEDURE AND THE ABOVE LISTED ITEMS (1–9).
I AM SATISFIED WITH THE EXPLANATION.

_____

Patient or person authorized to sign for patient.

Date _____

Witness _____

APPENDIX C: PHALLOPLASTY CONSENT

Informed consent—agreement for female-to-male gender confirmation surgery (phalloplasty, scrotoplasty, glansplasty, possible urethral lengthening, vaginectomy, possible placement of a suprapubic tube, and placement of skin graft or substitute to the flap donor site)

Instructions

This informed consent document has been prepared to inform you of female-to-male gender confirmation surgery (phalloplasty, scrotoplasty, glansplasty, possible urethral lengthening, vaginectomy, possible placement of a suprapubic tube, and placement of a skin graft or skin substitute to the flap donor site), its risks, as well as alternative treatments. It is important that you read this information carefully and completely. Please initial each page, indicating that you have read the page, and sign the consent for surgery as proposed by Loren S. Schechter, MD.

Informed consent documents are used to communicate information about the proposed surgical treatment of a disease or condition along with disclosure of risks and alternative forms of treatment(s). The informed consent process defines principles of risk disclosure that should generally meet the needs of most patients in most circumstances.

However, informed consent documents should not be considered all inclusive in defining other methods of care and risks encountered. Informed consent documents are not intended to define or serve as the standard of medical care. Standards of medical care are determined on the basis of all of the facts involved in an individual case and are subject to changes as scientific knowledge and technology advance and as practice patterns evolve.

Introduction

Female-to-male gender confirmation surgery is a surgical procedure to transform female anatomy into male anatomy. This surgery involves a phalloplasty (construction of the penis with a radial forearm flap or anterolateral thigh flap [ALT]), scrotoplasty (construction of the scrotum by conversion of the labia majora), glansplasty (shaping of the tip of the penis), vaginectomy (removal of the vagina), possible urethral lengthening and possible placement of a suprapubic tube, and placement of a skin graft or skin substitute on the flap donor site.

Alternative Treatments

Alternative forms of care consist of not undergoing surgery. Alternative types of surgery involve the creation of a penis using other tissues (for example, tissue from the back [MLD or musculocutaneous latissimus dorsi flap], performance of a metoidioplasty ["clitoral lengthening"]), or performance of a phalloplasty without urethral lengthening. Risks and potential complications are associated with alternative forms of treatment that involve surgery.

1. I,_____, hereby
authorize Loren S. Schechter, MD and such assistants and/or designees as may be selected to perform any or all of the following operations intended to transform female anatomy into male anatomy: phalloplasty (construction of the penis with a radial forearm flap or ALT), scrotoplasty

(construction of the scrotum by conversion of the labia majora), glansplasty (shaping of the tip of the penis), vaginectomy (removal of the vagina), possible urethral lengthening and possible placement of a suprapubic tube, and placement of a skin graft or skin substitute on the flap donor site.

2. This operation has been explained to me by Dr Loren S. Schechter, and I understand the nature and consequences of the procedure. I understand that during the course of the operation and/or medical treatment, unforeseen conditions could become apparent that may necessitate an extension of the original procedures or different procedures than those set forth above. I therefore authorize and request that Dr Loren S. Schechter and his assistants and/or designees perform such surgical procedures or render such medical treatments as are necessary and desirable in the exercise of professional judgment. The authority granted under this paragraph shall extend to treating the conditions that are both known and unknown to Dr Schechter at the time the operation is begun.

I also understand that it is impossible for a surgeon to disclose every conceivable risk, however remote. Although good results are expected, complications cannot be anticipated; therefore, there can be no guarantee either expressed or implied, as to the result of this surgery because the practice of medicine is not an exact science. Every surgical procedure involves a certain amount of risk, and it is important that you understand the risks involved with female-to-male gender reassignment surgery. Although most patients do not experience the following complications, you should discuss each of them with Dr Schechter to make sure that you understand the possible consequences of female-to-male gender reassignment surgery. The following points have been made specifically clear and are intended to provide information:

A. Scars result from any surgical procedure, but efforts are made to conceal or make them as inconspicuous as possible. Excessive scarring can occur. In rare cases, abnormal scars may result. Scars may be unattractive and of different color than the surrounding skin. Additional treatments including surgery may be necessary to treat abnormal scarring.

B. Signs of inflammation, such as tenderness, swelling, and discoloration (redness or black and blueness), occur that may last for several weeks or until the wound is completely healed. Residual swelling and redness can last a year or more.

C. Skin sensation: Numbness in or around the operative site may occur and may persist for an indefinite period of time. Occasionally this may be permanent. Numbness may also occur in the hands, arms, or legs due to the position of the body during surgery. This may or may not be permanent.

D. Infection may occur. Should an infection occur, treatment including antibiotics or additional surgery may be necessary.

E. Bleeding is possible during or after surgery. Should postoperative bleeding occur, it may require emergency treatment to drain accumulated blood (hematoma) or blood transfusion. I consent to the administration of whole blood or blood components. It has been explained to me that there is the possibility of ill effects including, but not limited to, infection and other diseases resulting from the administration of blood or blood components. I acknowledge and agree that neither the doctor nor the Hospital provides any guarantee nor warranty with respect to the blood or blood components. Should blood transfusion be required—you will be responsible for this additional cost.

F. Delayed healing: Wound disruption or delayed wound healing is possible. Some areas may not heal normally and/or may take a long time to heal. Some areas of the skin may die. This may require frequent dressing changes or further surgery to remove the nonhealed tissue. Unintentional interruption of blood supply to a flap, skin graft, or part of the operated area may result in its loss. Smokers have a greater risk of skin loss and wound-healing complications.

G. Seroma: Fluid accumulations infrequently occur. Should this problem occur, it may require additional procedures for drainage of fluid.

H. Asymmetry (noticeable difference in the size and shape) between the 2 sides of the operated area may result when both right and left sides are operated on.

I. Rectal injury: Inadvertent entry into the rectum may occur that could necessitate immediate closure of the opening, and the immediate or later creation of a colostomy (exteriorization of the colon in order that waste does not pass through the rectum).

J. Urethral, bladder, intestinal injury: Inadvertent entrance into the urethra, urinary bladder, or peritoneal cavity is a possibility and could cause later scar contracture or other unforeseeable problems in the future. A suprapubic tube may be placed during surgery.

K. Urethral fistula: A hole, or opening, of the newly created urethra may occur. This may require placement of a catheter or additional procedures.

L. Stenosis: Shortening or constriction of the newly made urethra or penis may occur and require additional procedures or use of urinary catheters.

M. Blood clots: Although rare, embolism from a blood clot may happen, which could result in death.

N. Allergic reactions: In rare cases, local allergies to tape, suture material, or topical preparations have been reported. Systemic reactions, which are more serious, may occur to drugs used during surgery and prescription medicines. Allergic reactions may require additional treatment.

O. Pain: Chronic pain may occur very infrequently from nerves becoming trapped in scar tissue.

P. Other: You may be disappointed with the results of surgery. Infrequently, it is necessary to perform additional surgery to improve your results. In addition, completely unpredictable and unusual complications, although extremely rare, including even death may occur. I understand that because of the nature of the above procedures, it is impossible to predict all the possible psychiatric and physiologic results. Some of the possible complications explained to me that can be involved in these procedures include in addition to those set forth above but not by way of limitation, are the following: severe loss of blood, infection, cardiac arrest, poor cosmetic results, permanent pain and discomfort, adverse affects from anesthesia, and psychiatric disorders.

Additional Surgery Necessary

Should complications occur, additional surgery or other treatments may be necessary. Even though risks and complications occur infrequently, the risks cited are particularly associated with female-to-male gender confirmation surgery.

1. I understand this operation is totally irreversible, and that I no longer will be able to have intercourse as a female or to conceive children. I also understand that Dr Loren S. Schechter does not guarantee any sexual pleasure or function as a result of the above stated procedures.

2. I consent to the administration of such anesthetics as may be considered necessary or advisable by the physician or anesthetist responsible for this service. There is the possibility of complications, injury, and even death from all forms of surgical anesthesia or sedation.

3. I consent to be photographed before, during, and after treatment, and I understand that these photographs are the visual part of my clinical record and are the property of Dr Loren S. Schechter, and may be published in scientific journals and/or shown for professional reasons. I hereby authorize Dr Loren S. Schechter and his assistants and/or his designees to use preoperative, intraoperative, and postoperative photographs, videotapes, and/or voice recordings for professional medical purposes deemed appropriate including, but not limited to, showing these images on public or commercial television, electronic digital networks, for purposes of medical education, patient education, lay publication, or during lectures to medical or lay groups. I understand that I will not be entitled to monetary payment or any other consideration as a result of any use of these images and/or my interview. I waive any right or option to inspect or approve the finished product or advertising or other copy that may be used along with the photographs, videotape, and voice recordings. I hereby grant Dr Loren S. Schechter the unlimited right to use such photographs, videotapes, and/or voice recordings as he deems appropriate, at his sole discretion.

4. For purposes of advancing medical education, I consent to the admittance of observers in the operating room. I have been advised, and I agree, that the surgical operation may be performed by a team of doctors including one or more attending doctors, residents, and medical students.

5. I consent to additional practitioners performing the procedure, or important aspects of the procedure, different from those now contemplated, whether or not arising from presently unforeseen conditions, whom Dr Schechter and/or his assistants and/or designees may consider necessary or advisable in the course of this operation.

6. I consent to the disposal of any tissue, medical devices, or body parts that may be removed.

7. I have been informed by Dr Loren S. Schechter that there are separate fees for surgical, medical, psychological, and anesthesia services as well as hospital fees. Additional costs may occur should complications develop from the surgery. Charges for secondary surgery or revisionary surgery would be your responsibility.

8. I certify that I have read and fully understand the above consent and agreement, which has been preceded by explanations by Dr Loren S. Schechter. I also certify that I have read and understand Dr Schechter's standard form letter regarding Gender Confirmation Surgery. His explanations in no way vary from the contents of this consent statement or his form letter and are understood by me. I agree not to revoke, limit, or alter this consent.

I fully understand all of the above, and I am satisfied with the explanation. I have no further questions. It has been explained to me in a way that I understand the treatment to be undertaken, the alternative methods of treatment, and the risks to the treatment. I authorize Loren S. Schechter, MD and his assistants and/or designees to perform any or all of the procedures discussed in this female-to-male gender confirmation surgery consent.

Patient_____

Date_____

Witness_____

In order to signify that you have read and understood the female-to-male gender confirmation surgery consent form, please complete the questionnaire.

Please list three possible complications of surgery:

1. _____

2. _____

3. _____

Please write in your own handwriting, "I have read and understood the female-to-male gender confirmation surgery consent form, and all of my questions have been fully answered" in the space provided below.

_____

_____

_____

Complete the following sentence found within the consent form:

"Should complications occur, _____."

Patient_____

Date_____

Witness_____

UNIVERSITY ❀
PLASTIC SURGERY

   In order to signify that you have been given all the information regarding your surgery, please complete the following questionnaire

   Please list 3 possible complications of surgery:

1. _____

2. _____

3. _____

   In order to signify that you have been given and have understood the possible complications of your surgery, please write in your own handwriting, "I have been educated on the risks, benefits, options, and alternatives for my surgery and all of my questions have been answered."

_____
_____
_____
_____
_____
_____

Patient:_____
Date:_____
Witness:_____

* This is attached to each of the consent forms

APPENDIX D: PREOPERATIVE AND POSTOPERATIVE INSTRUCTIONS

Preoperative instructions

In order to help you understand Dr Schechter's requirements, the following information is provided as a guideline only. Specific recommendations regarding your care will be made by Dr Schechter.

Patients' weight and gender confirmation surgery

Certain risks and complications of surgery are increased in people who are overweight or obese. In people who are morbidly obese, surgery will not be performed. In those individuals who are overweight, but not morbidly obese, the operation may be very difficult, and the final result may be compromised. The decision as to whether or not surgery will be performed will be determined by Dr Schechter.

Hormones and other drugs

Hormones should be discontinued 2 weeks before surgery. They may be resumed after surgery, once you are walking. Other medications which may cause prolonged bleeding should be discontinued before surgery. Specific questions regarding medications will be addressed by Dr Schechter before surgery.

Examples of medications to avoid before and after surgery:

Aspirin and aspirin-containing products

Ibuprofen and nonsteroidal anti-inflammatory medications (NSAIDs)

Herbal supplements and medications

Certain vitamins (check with Dr Schechter)

Anticoagulants/blood thinners, such as Coumadin/warfarin, Plavix, and Lovenox

Smoking

Smoking can result in poor healing, bad scars, and death of grafts and flaps. Surgery will not be performed in people who are smoking.

Postoperative instructions

What to Wear

Dark, loose fitting clothing is best; you should avoid tight elastic straps at the groin region.

Activity Restrictions

For the first 6 weeks after surgery, your activity will be limited. Limited activity means no heavy lifting (less than 10 pounds) or strenuous exercise. Six weeks after surgery, you may resume your usual activities.

Travel

If you are traveling to Chicago, you will be requested to stay in the area following discharge from the hospital. Specifics regarding length of stay will be reviewed by Dr Schechter.

APPENDIX E: POSTOPERATIVE VAGINOPLASTY INSTRUCTIONS

Following surgery, you will remain in bed for approximately 5 days. During this time, you will have a dilator in the vagina, a catheter in your bladder, and drains in the buttocks area.

While in the hospital, you will receive pain medication, an antibiotic, and a blood thinner. Additional medication, such as a stool softener and sleeping pill, may be prescribed.

Approximately 5 days after surgery, the dressing will be changed, and the vaginal dilator, urinary catheter, and drains may be removed. At this time, packing may be placed in the vagina. Dr Schechter will instruct you as to when to begin dilating. Specific instructions will depend upon your particular surgery (ie, penile inversion, use of skin graft, or intestinal vaginoplasty).

When you first get out of bed, you may be lightheaded. Lightheadedness is normal and tends to subside after a day or 2. The nurses will help you get out of bed and shower.

Following discharge from the hospital, you will have prescriptions for medications. These prescriptions will include a pain medication and stool softener. In addition, you may be prescribed a blood thinner. Our office will give you a date to see Dr Schechter following surgery.

APPENDIX F: POSTOPERATIVE CHEST SURGERY INSTRUCTIONS

After surgery, you will have an elastic wrap around your chest. This elastic wrap will remain in place until you are seen in Dr Schechter's office, typically about 4 to 6 days after surgery. In addition, you will have a drain (plastic tube) on each side of your chest. The nurses will instruct you in care of the drain. It is important to record the amount of output from the drain 2 to 3 times each day. The amount of drainage will be used to determine when the tubes are removed (done in the office).

After surgery, you will be discharged with pain medication, an antibiotic, a stool softener, and an anti-nausea medication.

You will be able to bathe, but not shower, until the dressings are removed. In addition, limit your lifting to less than 10 to 15 pounds and sleep with 2 pillows behind your head and back for the first week or so after surgery.

Following discharge from the hospital, you will be seen in Dr Schechter's office for follow-up care.

After your bandages are changed in Dr Schechter's office, you will apply an antibiotic ointment (such as bacitracin) 2 to 3 times each day to the nipples and areolae.

APPENDIX G: POSTOPERATIVE METOIDIOPLASTY INSTRUCTIONS

After surgery, you will have 2 urinary catheters: (1) a suprapubic tube (catheter in the bladder surgically placed in the lower abdominal region) and (2) a catheter in your penis (transurethral catheter). You will have bandages placed during surgery that will be changed before you leave the hospital.

While in the hospital, you will receive intravenous antibiotics, pain medication, and blood thinners, and you will wear compression boots on your legs. You will begin eating the day after surgery. Some people may experience nausea after surgery, and you will have medication available to help treat this.

Approximately 2 days after surgery, the bandages will be changed, and you will be able to shower. You will wear loose-fitting underwear with a gauze pad, because you will likely have some drainage. In addition, you will apply antibiotic ointment to your penis 2 times each day.

You will be discharged from the hospital with pain medication, a stool softener, antibiotics, and, possibly, a blood thinner. Your specific medications will be determined before leaving the hospital. In addition, you will receive instructions regarding care and maintenance of your suprapubic tube.

After approximately 3 weeks, the catheter will be removed from your penis. You may begin urinating through your penis, although the suprapubic catheter will likely remain in place until you have been consistently voiding. The suprapubic catheter will be removed following evaluation of your urethra.

Following discharge from the hospital, you will be seen in Dr Schechter's office for follow-up care.

APPENDIX H: POSTOPERATIVE PHALLOPLASTY INSTRUCTIONS

After surgery, you will be in the surgical intensive care unit (ICU). During that time, the nurses will monitor the blood flow to your penis with a handheld Doppler (a pencil-like device that listens to the artery in the penis). Your penis will be positioned upright with gauze bandages. In addition, you will have a suprapubic tube (catheter in the bladder surgically placed in the lower abdominal region) and a catheter in the penis (transurethral catheter). There will be a dressing on your forearm called a wound vac. This dressing consists of a foam sponge connected to a suction machine and it will be changed after 4 to 5 days and then every 2 to 3 days thereafter. You will receive intravenous antibiotics, pain medication, and blood thinners, and you will wear compression boots on your legs. You will begin drinking liquids a day or so after surgery. Some people may experience nausea after surgery, and you will have medication available to help treat this.

Following your stay in the ICU, you will transition to a surgical room. The nurses will continue to listen to the blood flow in your penis with the use of the Doppler, although less frequently than when in the ICU. You will begin to eat regular food and transition to oral medications (medication taken by mouth). You will also begin gentle therapy to assist with range of motion of your elbow, wrist, and fingers.

You will likely remain in bed for 5 to 7 days after surgery—when you first get out of bed, you may be a bit lightheaded. This lightheadedness is normal and will subside after a day or 2. In addition, you will wear surgical underwear to help support your penis—the penis should rest upwards, against your abdomen. When you are back in bed, you can place a rolled washcloth under your penis for support.

Approximately 2 to 3 weeks after surgery, if Integra was placed on your forearm donor site, you will return to surgery for a skin graft to be placed on your forearm. A wound vac will be placed for approximately 3 to 4 days, and there will be a bandage on your thigh (from where the skin graft was harvested).

After the wound vac has been changed on your forearm, you will begin every other day dressing changes to your forearm with an antibiotic ointment, gauze, and an Ace wrap.

You may be discharged from the hospital with pain medication, a stool softener, blood thinner, and antibiotics. The specific medications will be determined before leaving the hospital.

After approximately 3 weeks, the catheter will be removed from your penis. You may begin urinating through your penis, although the suprapubic catheter will remain in place. The suprapubic catheter will be removed following evaluation of your urethra.

Following discharge from the hospital, you will be seen in Dr Schechter's office for follow-up care.

Index

Printed and bound by CPI Group (UK) Ltd, Croydon, CR0 4YY

08/05/2025

01864758-0001